Competency Based

PHARMACOLOGY

Manual for MBBS Students

As per the latest
CBME Guidelines |
Competency Based Undergraduate Curriculum
for the Indian Medical Graduate

Name of the Student ....

Roll No. ....

Date of Admission ....

Mobile No. ....

E-mail ....

Competency Based
PHARMACOLOGY
Manual for MBBS Students

As per the latest
CBME Guidelines |
Competency Based Undergraduate Curriculum
for the Indian Medical Graduate

Arvind Yadav MD, ACME, MNAMS

Professor, Department of Pharmacology
Co-coordinator, Medical Education Unit (MEU)
Member Secretary, Institutional Ethics Committee
Geetanjali Medical College and Hospital, Udaipur, Rajasthan

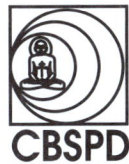

CBSPD

CBS Publishers & Distributors Pvt Ltd

New Delhi • Bengaluru • Chennai • Kochi • Kolkata • Lucknow • Mumbai
Hyderabad • Jharkhand • Nagpur • Patna • Pune • Uttarakhand

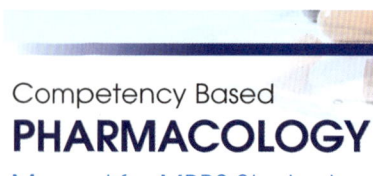

Competency Based
PHARMACOLOGY
Manual for MBBS Students

As per the latest
CBME Guidelines |
Competency Based Undergraduate Curriculum
for the Indian Medical Graduate

ISBN: 978-93-90709-96-0

First Edition: 2021
Reprint: 2022, 2023, 2024

Published by Satish Kumar Jain and produced by Varun Jain for

CBS Publishers & Distributors Pvt Ltd
4819/XI Prahlad Street, 24 Ansari Road, Daryaganj, New Delhi 110 002, India.
Ph: 23289259, 23266861   Website: www.cbspd.com
                                e-mail: delhi@cbspd.com

Corporate Office: 204 FIE, Industrial Area, Patparganj, Delhi 110 092
Ph: 011-4934 4934   Fax: 011-4934 4935   e-mail: publishing@cbspd.com; publicity@cbspd.com

Branches

- **Bengaluru:** Seema House 2975, 17th Cross, K.R. Road, Banasankari 2nd Stage, Bengaluru 560 070, Karnataka, India.
  Ph: +91-80-26771678/79   Fax: +91-80-26771680   e-mail: bangalore@cbspd.com
- **Chennai:** 7, Subbaraya Street, Shenoy Nagar, Chennai 600 030, Tamil Nadu, India.
  Ph: +91-44-26680620/26681266   Fax: +91-44-42032115   e-mail: chennai@cbspd.com
- **Kochi:** 42/1325, 26, Power House Road, Opp KSEB, Power House, Ernakulam 682 018, Kochi, Kerala, India.
  Ph: +91-484-4059061-65   Fax: +91-484-4059065   e-mail: kochi@cbspd.com
- **Kolkata:** 147, Hind Ceramics Compound, 1st Floor, Nilgunj Road, Belghoria, Kolkata 700056, West Bengal, India.
  Ph: +91-33-22891126, 22891127, 22891128   e-mail: kolkata@cbspd.com
- **Lucknow:** Basement, Khushnuma Complex, 7-Meerabai Marg (Behind Jawahar Bhawan), Lucknow-226 001, Uttar Pradesh, India.
  Ph: +0552-4000032   e-mail:tiwari.lucknowi@cbspd.com
- **Mumbai:** PWD shed, Gala No. 25/26, Ramchandra Bhatt Marg, Next to JJ Hospital Gate No. 2,
  OPP, Union Bank of India, Noorbaug, Mumbai-400009, Maharashtra, India.
  Ph: 022-66661880/89   Mob: 0-8424005858   e-mail: mumbai@cbspd.com

Representatives

• **Hyderabad**	0-9885175004	• **Jharkhand**	0-9811541605	• **Nagpur**	0-9421945513
• **Patna**	0-9334159340	• **Pune**	0-9923910676	• **Uttarakhand**	0-9716462459

Printed at: Gokul Offset Pvt. Ltd., D-159/A, Okhla Industrial Area, Phase-1, New Delhi, India

to
my beloved parents
Mrs Munni Devi and Mr Virendra Singh Yadav
and
my all respected teachers since childhood

Preface

Pharmacology is the science which deals with the drugs. Rational use of drugs/medicines is impossible without a proper understanding of their basic pharmacology, therefore this subject is the backbone of rational prescription in future for doctors. This manual is planned for the students of second MBBS as per new competency based medical education (CBME) of NMC. All the topics which are in skill or communication domain and already been defined by NMC in their curriculum (clinical pharmacy, experimental pharmacology and clinical pharmacology) are included in this manual. These include demonstration of various dosage forms including special drug delivery systems, dose calculations in special situations, routes of drugs administration through mannequins, computer assisting learning (CAL) for animal experiments, and various topics related to clinical pharmacology like drug promotion literature, p drug and essential medicine concept, ADR reporting and prescription writing and auditing including communication to patients about prescription.

Each exercise/practical in this manual has specific learning objectives related to that competency followed by teaching learning method and assessment. Relevant pictures/figures are used in the manual; not to promote them but to make topic more understanding and interesting for students who are visual learners.

Many places in medical colleges; much time are wasted in dictation of practical manual material compared to demonstration and as per new CBME curriculum, time for teaching pharmacology has also been reduced from 1.5 years to 1 year. So I thought to compile/write this manual as per new CBME based curriculum in pharmacology. I am not a big writer of book; I want to acknowledge the writer of many manuals and one specially running in Gujarat University since years, from which I have taken many important points because I considered them very much related to that topic and I also wish to acknowledge the authors of many theory and practical books running in India before implementation of CBME in pharmacology which helped me a lot.

Arvind Yadav

Acknowledgements

It is my pleasure to express gratitude to honourable Dr FS Mehta, Vice Chancellor, Geetanjali University, Rajasthan, for his constant inspiration and encouragement for writing this manual for the benefit of students so that they can focus more on learning and understanding part rather than writing part.

I want to thank my Head of Department, Dr Sangita Gupta, Geetanjali Medical College & Hospital, Udaipur, for her constant help, and guidance throughout the process of this manual.

This practical manual would be difficult without the knowledge gained by me from my teachers of UG and PG times Dr Varsha Patel, Professor and Head, Department of Pharmacology, Dr MK Shah Medical College & Research Centre, Ahmedabad; Dr Mira Desai, Professor and Head, Department of Pharmacology, Nootan Medical College and Research Centre, Visnagar; and Dr Chetna Desai, Professor and Head, Department of Pharmacology, BJ Medical College, Ahmedabad, from whom I learnt a lot about these topics. I thank them from the bottom of my heart.

Words defy me in expressing my deep sense of debt and gratitude to my staff members Dr Meenu Pichholiya, Associate Professor, Department of Pharmacology, GMCH, Udaipur, and Dr Haiya Sheth, Scientist D - ICMR PDC, Department of Clinical Pharmacology, Seth G.S. Medical College & K.E.M. Hospital, Mumbai, who unrelentingly helped me during the writing of this manual.

Words are too frail to express my deep feelings to my respected parents Mrs Munni Devi and Mr Virendra Singh for their unending affection, constant encouragement and invaluable help without whose blessings it would not have been possible for the present work to see the light of the day.

No words can express my gratitude and thanks to my lovely wife Dr Savita Choudhary without whose encouragement and strength this manual would not have taken its present shape. I also want to thank my sweet little kids Avi and Aashvi for making my world brighter while doing this work.

Lastly I want to thank CBS publishing team without which my efforts would not have been possible.

I am also thankful to CBS Publishers & Distributors. I would like to put on record the sincere efforts of Mr YN Arjuna (Senior Vice President Publishing, Editorial and Publicity), and his team comprising Ms Ritu Chawla (GM Production), Mr Parmod Kumar (DTP operator) and Mr Rohan (Graphic designer), for bringing out the book in the present form.

Arvind Yadav

CERTIFICATE

This is to certify that Mr/Ms _____ has

satisfactorily completed/not completed the practical work in Clinical Pharmacy, Experimental Pharmacology

and Clinical Pharmacology during the period from _____

to _____

Place:

Date:

_____

Signature of Head of the Department with Seal

(Department of Pharmacology)

Contents

Preface   *vii*

No.	Competency	Page no.	Date	Signature
	Clinical Pharmacy	**1**		
1.	PH1.9 Describe nomenclature of drugs, i.e. generic, branded drugs	1		
2.	PH2.1 Demonstrate understanding of the use of various dosage forms (oral/local/parenteral; solid/liquid) PH1.3 Enumerate and identify drug formulations and drug delivery system-**I (Solid Dosage Forms)**	6		
3.	PH2.1 Demonstrate understanding of the use of various dosage forms (oral/local/parenteral; solid/liquid) PH1.3 Enumerate and identify drug formulations and drug delivery system-**II (Liquid Dosages forms)**	16		
4.	PH2.1 Demonstrate understanding of the use of various dosage forms (oral/local/parenteral; solid/liquid) PH1.3 Enumerate and identify drug formulations and drug delivery system-**III (Inhalational dosage forms)**	26		
5.	PH2.1 Demonstrate understanding of the use of various dosage forms (oral/local/parenteral; solid/liquid) PH1.3 Enumerate and identify drug formulations and drug delivery system-**IV (Newer drug delivery systems)**	30		
6.	PH2.2 Prepare oral rehydration solution from ORS packet and explain its use	36		
7.	PH2.3 Demonstrate the appropriate setting up of an intravenous drip in a simulated environment	41		
8.	PH1.12 Calculate the dosage of drugs using appropriate formulae for an individual patient, including children, elderly and patient with renal dysfunction PH2.4 Demonstrate the correct method of calculation of drug dosage in patients including those used in special situations	47		
	Experimental Pharmacology	**52**		
9.	Introduction to experimental pharmacology	52		
10.	PH4.1 Administer drugs through various routes in a simulated environment using mannequins	56		
11.	PH4.2 Demonstrate the effects of drugs on blood pressure (vasopressor and vaso-depressors with appropriate blockers) using computer aided learning	63		

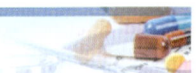

No.	Competency	Page no.	Date	Signature
	Clinical Pharmacology	**71**		
12.	PH1.64 Describe overview of drug development, Phases of clinical trials and Good Clinical Practice	71		
13.	PH1.10 Describe parts of a correct, complete and legible generic prescription. Identify errors in prescription and correct appropriately PH3.1 Write a rational, correct and legible generic prescription for a given condition and communicate the same to the patient	75		
14.	PH3.2 Perform and interpret a critical appraisal (audit) of a given prescription.	86		
15.	PH3.3 Perform a critical evaluation of the drug promotional literature	93		
16.	PH1.6 Describe principles of Pharmacovigilance and ADR reporting systems PH1.7 Define, identify and describe the management of adverse drug reactions (ADR) PH3.4 To recognise and report an adverse drug reaction	101		
17.	PH3.5 To prepare and explain a list of P-drugs for a given case/condition	111		
18.	PH3.6 Demonstrate how to optimize interaction with pharmaceutical representation to get authentic information of drugs	121		
19.	PH3.7 Prepare a list of essential medicines for a healthcare facility	125		
20.	PH3.8 Communicate effectively with a patient on the proper use of prescribed medication PH5.1 Communicate with the patient with empathy and ethics on all aspects of drug use PH5.2 Communicate with the patient regarding optimal use of (a) drug therapy, (b) devices and (c) storage of medicines PH5.3 Motivate patients with chronic diseases to adhere to the prescribed management by the healthcare provider PH5.4 Explain to the patient the relationship between cost of treatment and patient compliance	130		
21.	PH1.8 Indentify and describe the management of drug interactions	134		
22.	Notes	139		

Annexures   *157*
    I Format of checklist for assessment   *157*
    II Abbreviations, weight and measures   *158*
    III National list of essential medicine (NLEM) *159*
Logbook   *180*

CLINICAL PHARMACY

COMPETENCY PH1.9

Describe nomenclature of drugs, i.e. generic, branded drugs

Objectives

At the end of this practical class, students shall be able to:
- Define pharmacy, clinical pharmacy and other relevant terms
- Enumerate sources of drugs
- Differentiate between brand name and generic name
- Explain importance of expiry date
- Enlist components of a label
- Differentiate between prescription drug and non-prescription drugs.

Domain: Knowledge and skill
Level: Shows how
Teaching learning methods: Small group discussion, demonstration
Aligning assessment methods: Written, viva voce
Number of procedure to be done independently for certification: None

Pharmacy

It is a science of identification, compounding and dispensing of drug including interpretation and evaluation of prescriptions. It also comprises collection, identification, purification, isolation, synthesis, standardization and quality control of medicinal substances. The large scale manufacture of drugs is called pharmaceutics.

Clinical Pharmacy

The American College of Clinical Pharmacy (ACCP) defines clinical pharmacy as an area of pharmacy concerned with the science and practice of rational medication use. It is an area where pharmacists provide optimal treatment approach for optimal patient care outcome with the help of specialized knowledge and judgement.

Pharmacist

He or she is a qualified person who is authorized to prepare and dispense different dosage forms of the drugs.

Pharmacognosy

It is the branch of pharmacology which deals with the knowledge of medicinal drugs obtained from plants or other natural origins.

Posology

It is a branch of pharmacology concerned with drug dosage and dosage regimen.

Dose

It is a quantity of the drug which produces desired therapeutic response in a recipient.

Drug

As per WHO a drug is a substance or product, which is used or intended to be used to modify or explore the physiological or pathological state for the benefit of the recipient.

NATURE AND SOURCES OF DRUGS

Drugs can be solid, liquid and gases in nature. Drugs are the chemical substances which are mostly organic in nature but inorganic compounds like ferrous compounds, antacids, etc. are also used in various conditions. Drugs

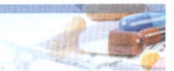

can be obtained naturally or they are semi-synthetically and synthetic derived. Nowadays most of the drugs used for treatment purpose are synthetically derived because of good quality in terms of safety, efficacy and they can be produced in large quantity as compared to natural sources which are limited.

Sr. No.	Drug sources	Examples
1.	Plants	Plants products may be alkaloids, glycosides, and some plant products like oils (castor oil, peppermint oil), gums (gum acacia), tannins (tincture catechu), and resins (Tolu balsum) are used to prepare various drug formulations. For example, morphine (papavarum somniferum), quinine (cinchona), digoxin (digitalis purpurea), atropine (atropa belladonna), etc.
2.	Animals	Heparin, antisera, vaccines and hormones like insulin, thyroxine, etc.
3.	Microorganism	Many antimicrobial agents like penicillin from fungus (Penicillium notatum), chloramphenicol from actinomycetes (streptomyces venezuele) , polymyxin B and bacitracin from bacteria (Bacillus group), etc.
4.	Minerals	Magnesium sulphate, aluminium hydroxide and silicate, ferrous sulphate, etc.
5.	Human derived	Immunoglobulins, HCG, etc. Nowadays many drugs are produced by recombinant DNA technology. For example, insulin, t-PA
6.	Synthetic	Majority of the drugs are now synthesized. For example, fluoroquinolones, ACE inhibitors, etc.

DRUG NOMENCLATURE

- **Chemical name:** It denotes the chemical constitution of a drug which is complex and difficult to use in prescriptions. For example, acetylsalicylic acid, ethyl alcohol, etc.
- **Non-proprietary (Generic) or official name:** It is the name which is decided by an expert committee and is accepted and understood internationally. It is given by the official bodies like United States Adopted Name (USAN) Council (USAN) or British Approved Name (BAN) Council and commonly known as International Non-proprietary Name (INN). The generic names have some elements for drug categorization representing their pharmacological classification. For example, 'caine' for local anaesthetics, 'pril' for ACE inhibitors, etc.
- **Proprietary (Brand) name:** It is the name chosen by the pharmaceutical company of the drug and this name is a copyright or registered name of the drug. These names are short and easy to remember. Brand names for a drug may vary country-wise and hence may not be recognized universally. One drug may have multiple brand names. For example, Calpol, Crocin, Dolo are the brand name for paracetamol.

Example: Nomenclature of single drug:
Chemical name: Acetylysalicylic acid
Generic name: Aspirin
Brand name: Ecospirin, Disprin

EXPIRY DATE OF MEDICINES

The manufacturing date of medicines is stamped on the outer carton as well as on the bottle or strip. A unique batch number or lot number characterizes the manufacturing date. The date of expiry is calculated from the production date and is also stamped below the manufacturing date. The period between two dates is called "life-period" or "shelf-life" of the drug. Life period of most of the drugs is between 1 and 5 years (Schedule P). The expiry date depends on the rate of decomposition of the medicinal product. The rate of decomposition depends on the temperature, relative humidity, light exposure and addition of preservatives. Preservatives of different types inhibit microbial growth and hence degradation and spoilage. Hence instructions on storage are given on the outer container and the inner packing. Expiry date of a preparation is decided after carrying out the primary, secondary and real time stability tests. Visible changes after expiry date of drugs can occur; like change in colour, consistency, friability and solubility in case of tablets and powders and fermentation, change in colour, taste and appearance of particulate matter (precipitation) in case of liquids may occur in drugs that are either not preserved

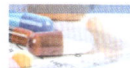

as per specifications or those which are expired. Liquid formulations are also less stable. Use of expired drugs can cause following effects:

- **Loss of efficacy:** Due to change in chemical composition which leads to decreased effect.
- **Adverse effects/toxicity:** Degradation products that are formed may be toxic. For example, epianhydrotetracycline is formed after expiry of tetracycline causes Fanconi's syndrome, adrenochrome from adrenaline is hepatotoxic, etc.
- **Contamination:** Bacterial and fungal contamination of the drug may occur. Use of this can lead to resistance.

Label

It is usually attached or printed on the container or strip and also on the outer carton. It provides useful information about the following:

1. The trade and generic name of the drug(s).
2. The type of formulation.
3. Ingredients of the preparation and their quantity.
4. The dosage instructions.
5. The manufacture and expiry date of the preparation.
6. Instructions for use of the preparation.
7. Precautions and warning, if any, with respect to the use of the drug.
8. Address of the manufacturer and the marketing agency of the drug.
9. Batch number, manufacturing license number and the MRP of the preparation.
10. Schedule of drug.

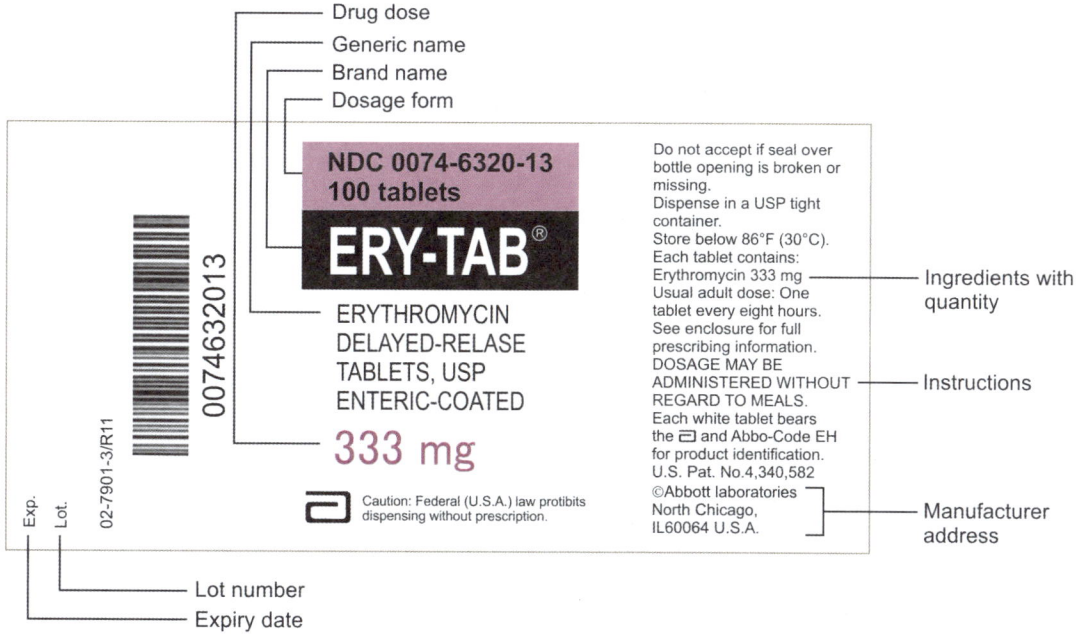

DRUG REGULATIONS

To regulate the import, manufacture, distribution and sale of drugs, the Government of India has formulated the Drugs and Cosmetic Act. Drugs Controller General of India (DCGI) and Food and Drug Administration (FDA) govern this act. The Drugs and Cosmetic Act classifies drugs as per safety, addiction liability and poisonous/non-poisonous nature into following categories:

1. **Over the counter drugs (non-prescription drugs):** They are considered to be relatively safe drugs, used for common ailments and can be sold over the counter without prescription. For example, paracetamol, antacids, laxatives, etc.
2. **Prescription drugs:** These are the drugs which as per the drug rules; must be sold in retail, only against a prescription issued to a patient by a registered medical practitioner. For example, all antibiotics.

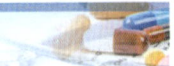

As per the Drugs and Cosmetic Rules in India; there are various schedules for the drugs. Few important are the following:

Schedule A: Gives the specimens of prescribed forms.

Schedule F and F (I): Give details of the standards of bacterial vaccines made from any microorganism pathogenic to man or other animals and also the vaccines made from other microorganisms which have any antigenic value.

Schedule G: Details the drugs to be labelled with the words "Caution—it is dangerous to take this preparation except under medical supervision".

Schedule H: Deals with drugs and medicines which must be sold by retail only when a prescription by registered medical practitioner is produced. Most drugs fall under this schedule.

Schedule P: Deals with the life period of drugs including combinations with other drugs. It gives period in months for which the drug is expected to retain its potency under the conditions of storage notified by licensing authority.

Schedule V: Gives details of standards for patent and proprietary medicines.

Schedule W: Gives the names of the drugs which shall be marketed under generic names only.

Schedule X: Gives the names of psychotropic drugs requiring special licenses for manufacture and sale.

Schedule Y: Specifies requirements and guidelines on clinical trials, import and manufacture of new drugs.

LET'S DO THIS

1. WHO definition of drug.

2. Write two drug sources name with example of each.

3. What are the advantages of drug prescribing by generic names?

4. What is schedule H?

_____

_____

_____

_____

_____

_____

5. Why we should not take expired drug?

_____

_____

_____

_____

_____

_____

6. What do you mean by shelf-life of the drug?

_____

_____

_____

_____

_____

_____

7. Write full form of the following:

DGCI: _____

FDA: _____

8. What are OTC drugs?

_____

_____

_____

_____

_____

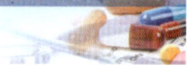

Date:

PRACTICAL 2

COMPETENCY

PH2.1: Demonstrate understanding of the use of various dosage forms (oral/local/parenteral; solid/liquid)

PH1.3: Enumerate and identify drug formulations and drug delivery system

Objectives

At the end of this practical class, students shall be able to:
- Explain concept of drugs and excipients in formulations
- Identify different solid oral dosage forms
- Identify different solid topical dosage forms
- State advantages and disadvantages of oral dosage forms
- Learn the correct method of using these dosage forms.

Domain: Skill and communication

Level: Shows how

Teaching learning methods: Small group discussion, DOAP

Aligning assessment methods: Skill assessment, viva voce

Number of procedure to be done independently for certification: None

Materials Needed

Sample of various oral dosage forms like tablet, capsule, powder, etc.

Dose

It is a quantity of the drug which produces desired therapeutic response in a recipient. Formulation: It is a recipe by which a drug is prepared. It contains active ingredients like drugs and other substances like excipients, vehicles, flavouring agents and preservatives.

Excipients

Pharmacologically inert substances added to the pharmaceutical preparation when a small quantity of the drug is present, to add bulk and give appearance to the tablet. These are also used to mask the unpleasant taste. For example, lactose, calcium lactase, starch, etc.

Vehicles

These are added in pharmaceutical preparations to dissolve or suspended the drugs, to make them better applicable (as in ointments) or more palatable (as in liquids). For example, sugar syrups, cherry syrup, petroleum jelly, etc. Binders: It binds the drug particles together in case of tablet.

Lubricants

It helps keep the tablet from sticking to the manufacturing machine.

Aqua

These are watery solutions of volatile oils or other aromatic substances in distilled water. For example, Aqua mentha preperatta.

Colouring Agents

These are harmless substances used for imparting colour to a dosage form. For example, Carmine, amaranth red (colouring agent used in tincture cardamom).

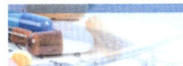

Flavouring Agents

Different flavours are used to mask nauseating and unpleasant taste of medicines. For example, spirit chloroformis.

Sweetening Agents

Different sweetening agents like sucrose are used to mask bad taste of syrups and elixirs; another saccharine which is a non caloric sweetener may be used in diabetics and obese patients. Aspartame is an artificial non-saccharide sweetener used as a sugar substitute in some foods and beverages.

Dosage form

These are the different drug formulations which are designed to make it possible to introduce a drug into the human body. Dosage forms are of different types; vary from a simple solution to very complex drug delivery systems. For example, solid dosage forms, liquid dosage forms, inhalational dosage forms, topical dosage forms and newer drug delivery systems.

A. Solid oral Dosage forms

The following are the most commonly used solid dosage forms as they provide a correct compact dosage, are portable, usually bland to taste and are convenient to market, store and administer. The oral forms should be swallowed with a full glass of water with the patient in upright posture.

Advantages of oral solid dosage forms
- Appropriate for any age of patient
- The most common, natural and easiest route of administration
- Safe, economical and convenient to the patient
- Patient can take it without any help (self-administered).

Disadvantages of oral solid dosage forms
- Delayed onset of action because absorption takes time
- Not suitable in emergency and for unconscious patients
- Not convenient for a patient with vomiting and diarrhoea
- Not suitable for uncooperative patients as children and infants.

1. Tablets

These contain unit dose of one or more powdered or granulated drugs that are prepared by compressing under heavy pressure or moulding methods into a round or disk-like shape suitable for swallowing. They are also available in triangular or cylindrical shapes. Tablets are the most popular as dosage forms.

The different types of tablets are:

Uncoated tablets: Tablets are having no coating. *Example:* Aspirin tablet.	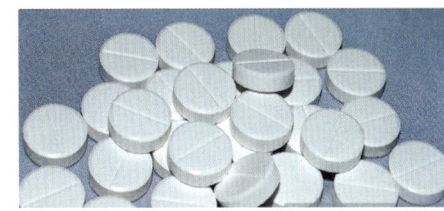
Coated tablets: The tablets are coated with one or more layers of mixtures of substances for a variety of reasons like protecting drug from air, moisture or light, etc. **Sugar coated tablets:** Coated with sugar to enhance palatability. *Example:* Tablet chloroquine, metronidazole. **Film coated tablets:** A transparent film is made up of cellulose-acetate and gelatin derivatives to mask the unpleasant taste. *Example:* Cefuroxime film coated tablet, diltiazem film coated tablet.	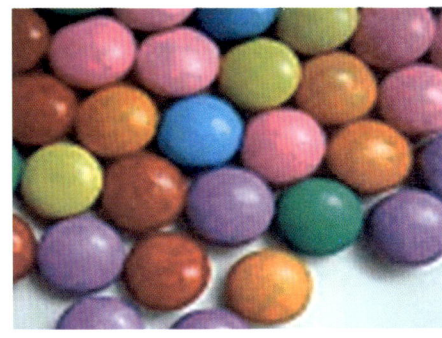

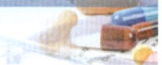

Enteric coated tablets (delayed-release): These single or multilayer coating intended to resist digestion by gastric acid but get disintegration in the alkaline medium of intestinal fluid. They should be taken as a whole in unbroken form. This is a suitable dosage forms for gastric irritant drugs administered by the oral route.
Example: Diclofen 25/50 (Diclofenac enteric coated tablet)

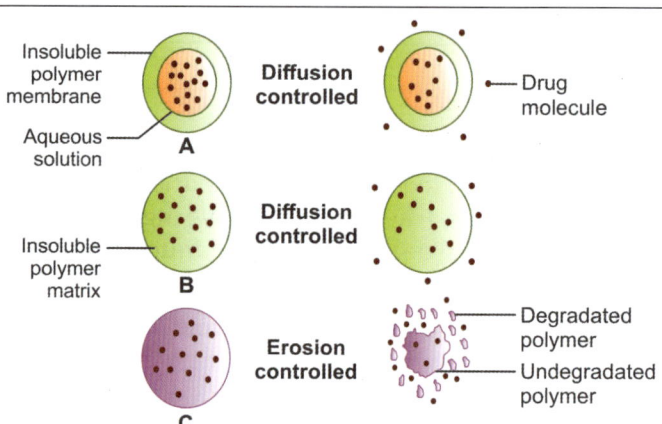

Sustained-release tablets (extended/prolonged-release tablets): Drug particles are coated with different types of inert resins so that each type of coating dissolves at different time intervals. On administration initially the drug is released rapidly to provide concentrations sufficient to cause desired response and then sustained release at a constant rate is sufficient for maintenance therapy for prolonged period. This lead to reduced frequency of administration and good patient compliance but these are more expensive than the conventional dosage forms.
Example: Diclonac-SR (Diclofenac sod. SR), Depin Retard (Nifedipine retard tablet).

Scored tablets: These tablets contain break marks or other markings on their surface so that they can be easily divided into smaller doses. Breaking in small pieces is not possible in un-scored tablets.

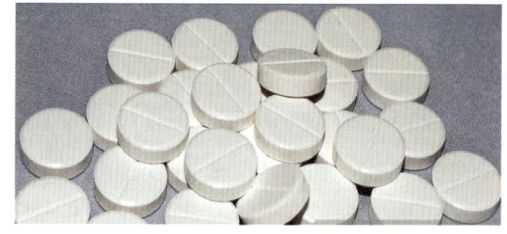

Dispersible tablets: These disintegrate rapidly in water and are intended to be dispersed in water before administration.
Example: Amoxicillin dispersible tablet.

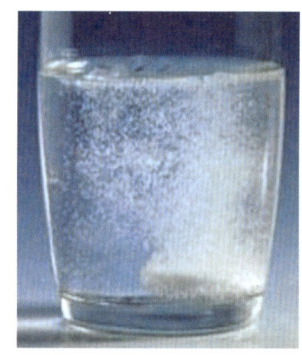

Effervescent tablets: These are uncoated tablets containing acidic substances, carbonates or bicarbonates which react rapidly in the presence of water to release carbon dioxide. They are intended to be dissolved or dispersed in water before administration. They mask the bad taste of the drug, carbon dioxide released may act as carminative and may also have a psychological effect on the patient.
Example: Gastica-fiz tablet.

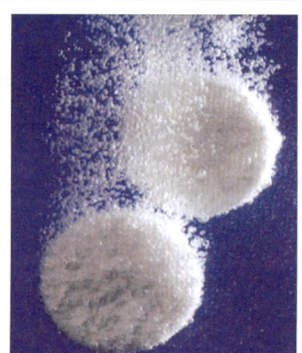

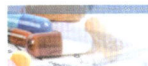
Tablets for use in the mouth

Chewable tablets: These are large tablets, usually pleasant tasting, that are meant to be chewed well before swallowing. Chewing provides disintegration in the mouth; so produces rapid effect after swallowing.
Example: Vit C, D_3 and K_2 tablets.

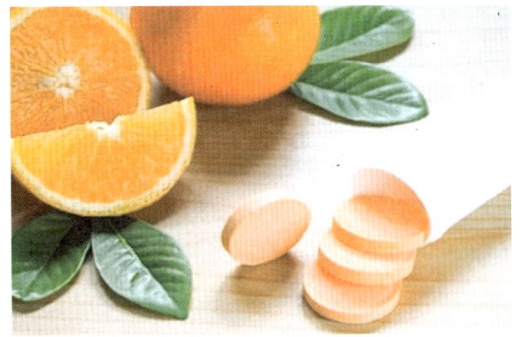

Sublingual or buccal or tablets: These are small, flat or oval tablets intended to be inserted in the buccal pouch or beneath the tongue where the active ingredients may be directly absorbed through the mucosa, into the systemic circulation.
Example: GTN, nitrates.

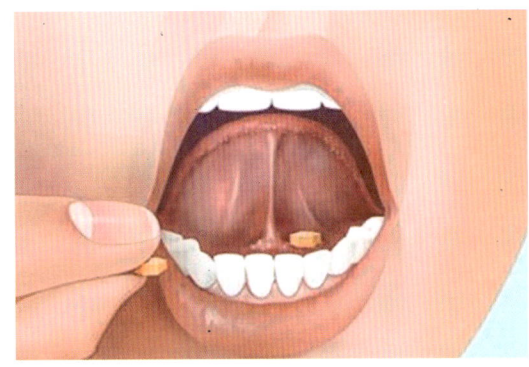

Lozenges or troches: These are flat, rounded or rectangular preparations kept in mouth till they dissolve. They temporarily produce high concentration of the drug in the oral cavity and are used to treat local conditions of the mouth or throat.
Example: Cough Lozenges (Strepsil)

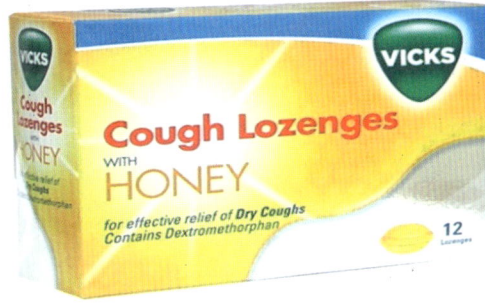

Mouth dissolving tablet (orally disintegrating tablets, ODTs): New generation formulation with advantages of both liquid and tablet forms. These are especially designed for dysphagic, geriatric, pediatric, bedridden, travelling and psychotic patients. They dissolve/disintegrate very fast when placed in mouth and no manual chewing is required like lozenges. They do not require water for its administration.
Example: Ondansatran, domperidone.

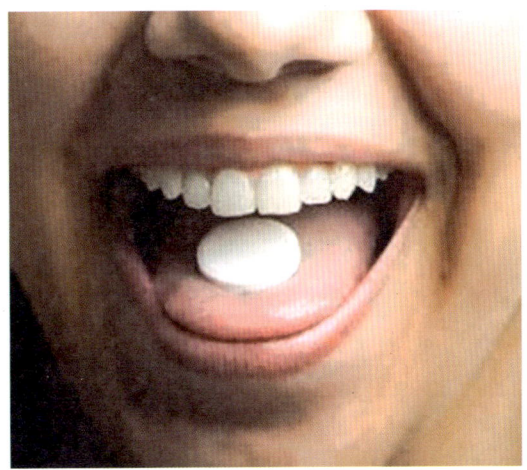

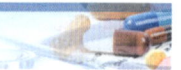

2. Capsules

These are small containers, usually made of gelatin. They may be hard or soft. They are available in different colours and are usually bland to taste. Solid, liquids and paste like consistency contents can be administered as capsules. They dissolve readily in the gastrointestinal tract (GIT).

Example: Tetracycline capsule, amoxicillin capsule, chloramphenicol capsule.

The different types of capsules are:

Hard capsule: Shells of two cylindrical sections are joined together in it which are made up of gelatin. Drug may be either in granules or powder form. *Example:* Tetracycline capsule	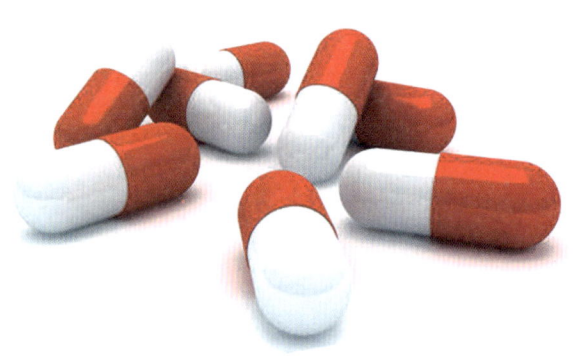
Soft capsule: Single shell of thick gelatin layer. Drug is in liquid form. *Example:* Cod liver oil	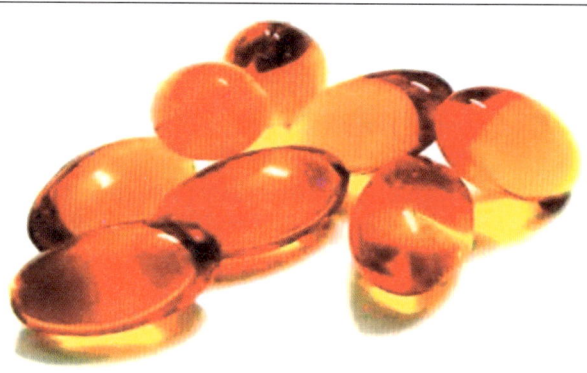
Modified-release capsules or spansules: These are designed to modify the rate, place or time of release of drug. They can be of delayed release type or sustained release type like tablets. *Example:* Ferrous sulfate, omeprazole etc.	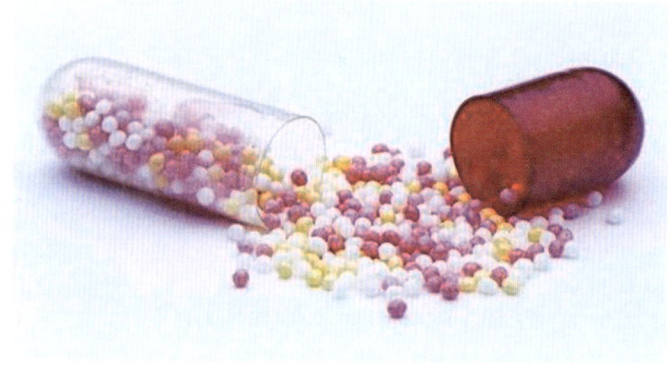

3. Powders

Powders are solid dosage form of drugs in a finely divided form and are mixed homogeneously. They are easy to dispense, can be weighed accurately and administered to children with great ease (with few exceptions). Unpleasant or unpalatable drugs cannot be dispensed in powder form.

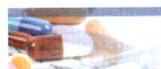

Simple powder: It contains only one ingredient in either crystalline form or amorphous form.
Example: Glucose power, aspirin powder

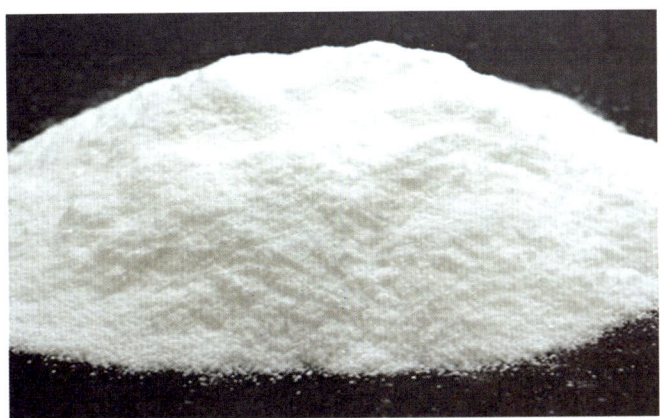

Compound powder: It contains two or more than two ingredients which are mixed together.
Example: ORS powder

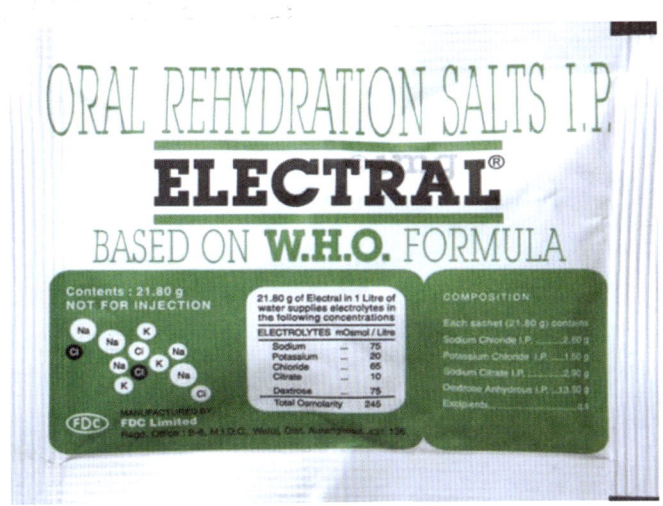

Granular effervescent powders: These powders contain drug with mixture of acid and alkali which after dissolving in water release carbon dioxide after reaction. It masks the bitter taste.
Example: ENO

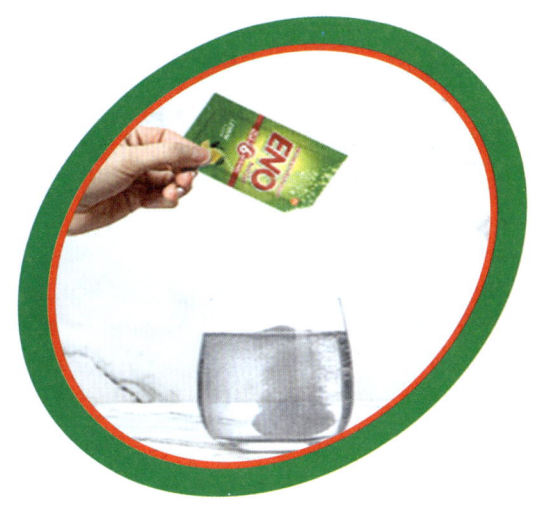

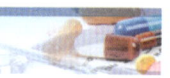

4. Granules

Granules are small irregular particles; 0.5–2 mm in diameter, aggregated together by a binding agent; often supplied in single dose sachets. Granulation allows addition of flavouring and colouring agents so as to make them palatable and attractive. Some are placed on the tongue and swallowed with water.
Example: Zinc granules, calcitriol

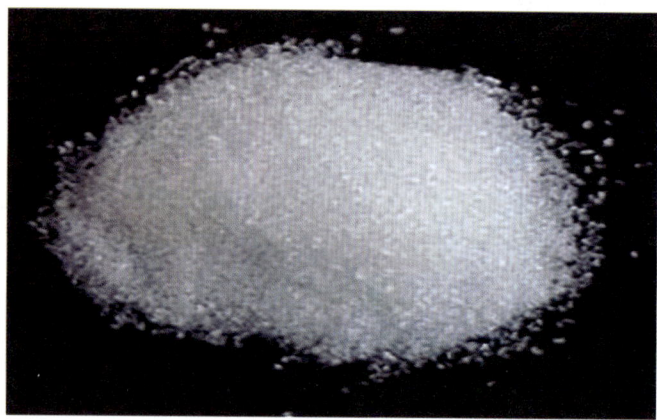

5. Cachet

Cachet provides an edible container like capsule. It consists of two concave pieces of wafer made of flour and water filled with drug and sealed tightly by moistening the margins and pressing firmly. It becomes soft, elastic and slippery when moistened with water and hence swallowed easily.
Example: Vit E and evening prime rose oil cachets.

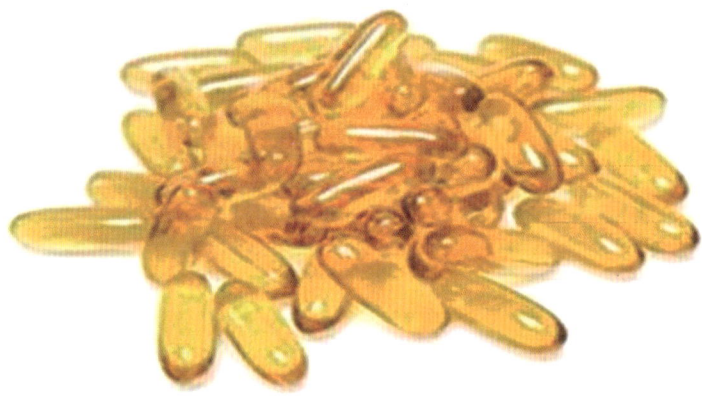

B. Solid Topical Dosage forms

Dusting powder: Powders intended for local use with no systemic effects.
Example: Neomycin powder, boric acid powder.
Plasters: Plasters are solid adhesive preparations applied to protect, soothe, and provide mechanical support and to lessen pain. They also bring medicament close to the skin.
Example: Johnson and Johnson, zinc oxide plaster
Pellets: These are sterile spheres formed by compression of the drug. They are implanted subcutaneously and form a depot from where drug is released slowly for a long duration. They are marketed in sterile vials.
Example: Testosterone pellets.

C. Other Solid Dosage forms

Suppositories

These are mixtures of drugs with a firm base that can be moulded in shapes suitable for insertion into cavity or orifice. They melt at body temperature and release medication which comes in contact with mucous membrane to produce mainly local effect.

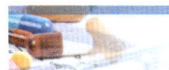

Rectal suppositories are cone or bullet shaped to be placed in rectum for the evacuation of the bowel before a radiological examination or as an enema alternative and constipation.

Example: Dulcolax suppositories for constipation

Vaginal suppositories (Pessaries) are conical or spherical to be placed in vagina to provide high local concentration of the drug at the site.

Example: Miconazole + Tinidazole antifungal vaginal pessaries

Urethral suppositories (bougies) are pencil shaped. They are supplied in aluminium foil and are usually lubricated with a water soluble jelly.

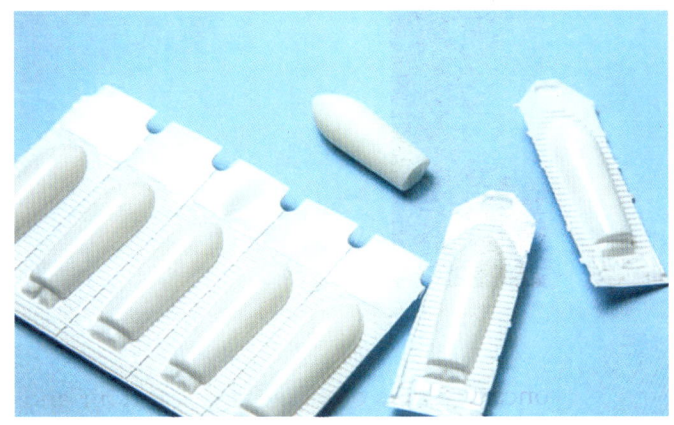 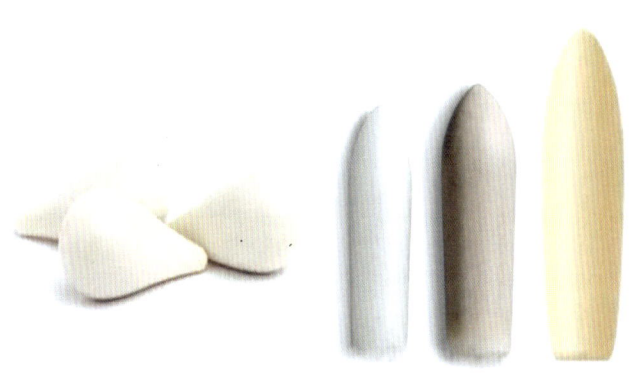

LET'S DO THIS

1. What are excipients?

_____

_____

_____

_____

_____

_____

2. a. Identify the type of tablet shown in given picture.
   b. What is the importance of marking over tablet?

_____

_____

_____

_____

_____

_____

_____

_____

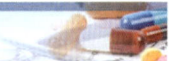

3. a. Identify the type of tablet shown in given picture.
   b. Write an example.

   _____

   _____

   _____

   _____

   _____

   _____

   _____

   _____

   _____

   _____

4. a. Identify the dosage form in this picture
   b. Write two difference between hard and soft capsules.

   _____

   _____

   _____

   _____

   _____

   _____

5. What are spansules?

   _____

   _____

   _____

   _____

   _____

6. Identify the dosage form and write two
   disadvantages of this dosage form.

   _____

   _____

   _____

   _____

   _____

   _____

7. Why does CO_2 release from effervescent tablets? What is the advantage of this mechanism?

_____

_____

_____

_____

_____

_____

8. Write one advantage and one disadvantage of sustained release tablet.

_____

_____

_____

_____

_____

_____

_____

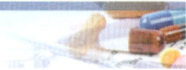

Date:

PRACTICAL 3

COMPETENCY

PH2.1: Demonstrate understanding of the use of various dosage forms (oral/local/parenteral; solid/liquid)

PH1.3: Enumerate and identify drug formulations and drug delivery

Objectives

At the end of the practical class, the student shall be able to:

- Identify and list the common liquid dosage forms used for topical or systemic routes.
- Enlist advantage and disadvantages of liquid oral dosage forms
- Demonstrate the steps for liquid topical dosage forms. For example, eyedrops, eardrops, nasal drops
- Differentiate between ampoule and vial.

Domain: Knowledge and communication

Level: Shows how

Teaching learning methods: Small group discussion, DOAP

Aligning assessment methods: Skill assessment, OSPE with checklist, viva voce

Number of procedure to be done independently for certification: None

Materials Needed

Sample of various liquid dosage forms like syrup, ointment, gel, vial, ampoule, eyedrops, nasal spray, etc.

The liquid dosage forms are prepared by dissolving active ingredients in aqueous or non-aqueous solvents and can be administered orally, parenterally or applied locally.

Advantages of Liquid Oral Dosage forms

1. Easy to administer in children and elderly.
2. Better absorbed and quickly effective.
3. Certain drugs may cause gastric pain when given in the dry form and hence are safer when administered as solution. For example, salts of potassium iodide and bromide.

Disadvantages of Liquid Oral Dosage forms

1. They are less stable
2. They have unpleasant taste
3. They are bulky and inconvenient to store and transport. Accidental breakage may cause loss of drug,
4. Dose administered may not be accurate, especially when household measures are used.

Liquid Oral Dosage forms

1. Solutions

These are clear homogenous liquid preparations containing one or more soluble chemicals dissolved in a solvent. Solutions can be used either internally or externally.

Elixirs

These are clear flavoured hydroalcoholic solutions of medicinal substances. They are usually less sweet and less viscous due to less sugar as compared to syrups

Example: Vitamin B-complex elixirs, cough elixers.

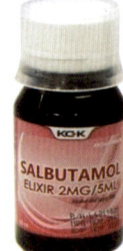

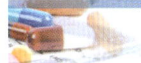

Syrup

Syrups are concentrated sucrose solution in water or other liquids. They may be simple (only purified water), medicated (active drug) or flavoured (aromatic or flavoured) for using as a vehicle. They contain high sugar and also more effective as compared to elixir. Syrups are commonly used for children.

Example: Cough and vitamin syrups.

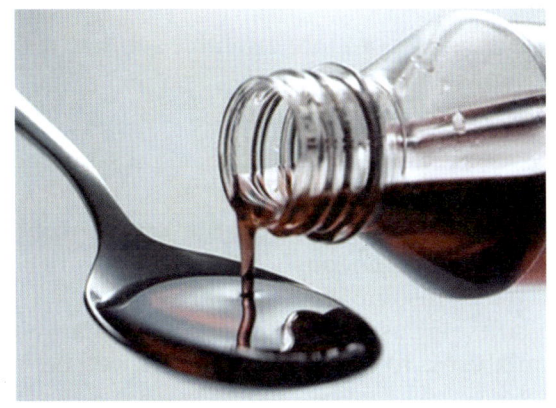

Linctus

These are viscous liquids containing the drug with some demulcents (menthol), sugar and alcohol intended to use for relief of cough. It has to be sipped and swallowed slowly without addition of water.

Example: Cough linctus.

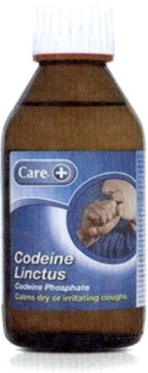

Tinctures

These are solutions prepared by extracting the active content from a crude drug. They can be obtained from vegetable material (alcoholic or hydroalcoholic) or from chemicals.

Example: Tinct. digitalis, tinct. belladonna.

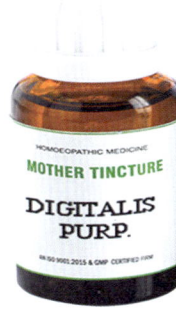

Oral drops

Drops are solutions, tinctures or mixtures of drug substances to be prescribed in small quantities intended to be used orally. Oral drops are mainly for paediatric use. They facilitate accurate dosing in infants. They may be solutions, suspensions or emulsions.

Example: Vitamin drops and enzyme drops.

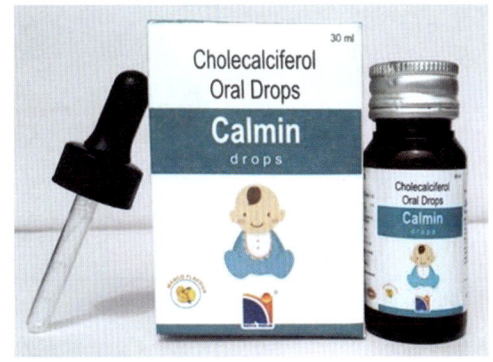

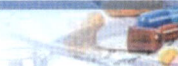

2. Suspensions

These contain one or more insoluble solid drugs dispersed in vehicle homogeneously with or without the help of suspending agent.

Example: Antidiarrhoeal mixture

Mixture

These are solid drugs, soluble or insoluble, dispersed homogeneously in vehicle meant for internal use. Insoluble particles are suspended by using suitable suspending agent (agar agar) and such mixture is to be labeled as 'shake well before use'.

Example: Antidiarrhoeal mixtures, Milk of magnesia, $MgSO_4$ mix, etc.

Mixture effective in and dispensed as single dose is known as draught.

Example: Cathartic mixture

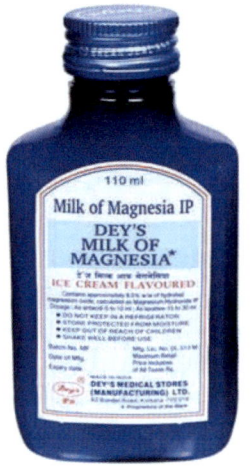

Emulsions

Emulsion is a mixture of two immiscible liquids, one of which is dispersed uniformly throughout the other with the help of emulsifying agent. The dispersed liquid is the discontinuous phase and the dispersion medium is known as the continuous phase. They are used orally to mask the unpleasant taste; absorption of drug is faster (finely divided phase increases total surface area).

Example: Cod liver oil emulsion, liquid paraffin emulsion, castor oil emulsion.

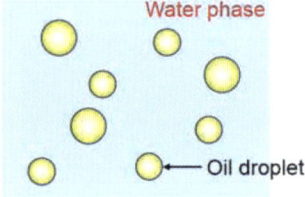
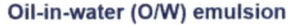
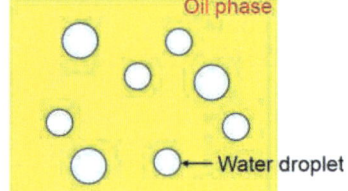

Oil-in-water (O/W) emulsion   Water-in-oil (W/O) emulsion

Magmas

These are bulky suspensions of poorly soluble substances in water. Since they are white liquids, they are also known as milks.

Example: Bentonite magma, aluminium hydroxide magma.

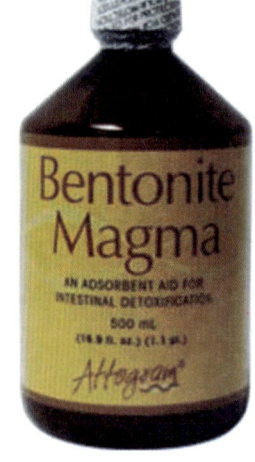

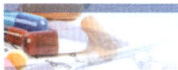

3. Dry mixtures for Solution

Agents having insufficient stability in aqueous solutions to meet extended shelf-life periods are provided as dry powders or granules for reconstitution with required quantity of purified water immediately before administration. Solutions are usually stable for 7–10 days after refrigeration.

Example: ORS powder, cephalexin dry syrup etc.

Liquid Topical Dosage forms

Liniments

They are liquid preparations intended for external application on unbroken skin by rubbing or inunction. They contain medicaments in a liniment base (vehicle) of a fixed oil or soap and water or alcohol. Usually it contains substances which are analgesic, rubifacient, mild astringent or counter irritant property.

Example: Turpentine methyl salicylate liniment, camphor liniment.

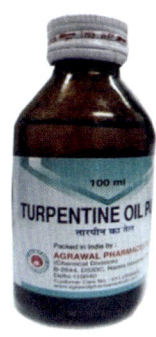

Lotions

They are liquid preparations meant for local application to the skin or mucous membrane without rubbing. They can be protective, emollient, cooling, cleansing, astringent, antipruritic and antiseptic depending on the type of content.

Example: Calamine lotion

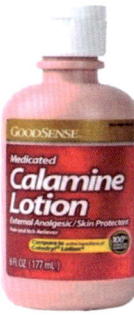

Ointments

They are semisolid preparation with a greasy base as vehicle for external application to skin and mucous membrane. They contain petroleum base like hard and soft paraffin or wool fat to produce emollient action and helps in keeping medicament in prolong contact.

Example: Chloramphenicol eye ointment, atropine eye ointment, nitroglycerine ointment.

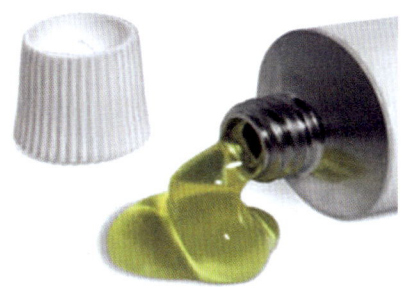

Pastes

They are semisolid preparations contain a non greasy base (hence washable). Paste does not melt at body temperature like ointments. They are prepared from some adhesive material like starch or a foaming agent like carboxymethyl cellulose. For example, zincs oxide pastes, toothpastes. They are applied to oozing surfaces and afford greater protection and more absorptive action than ointments; easy to apply and suitable for hairy parts. They act as vehicles in certain medications.

Example: Anhydrous benzoyl peroxide toothpaste.

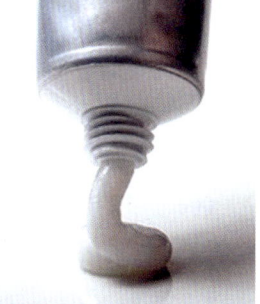

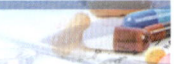

Creams

They are viscous liquid or semisolid emulsion which can be either oil in water or water in oil type. They may contain drug or other substances depending on the purpose. They may be applied to skin or mucous membrane.

Example: Betnovate cream, momate-F (Mometasone Furoate and Fusidic Acid cream).

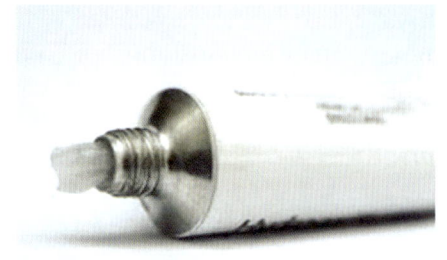

Gels

Drug is dissolved in a liquid and then dispersed in some gelling agent (soft gelatin). They are usually transparent preparation For example, lignocaine gel, ketoprofen 2% oral gel. However the term is also used for colloidal aqueous suspension of hydrated inorganic substances.

Example: Aluminium hydroxide gels.

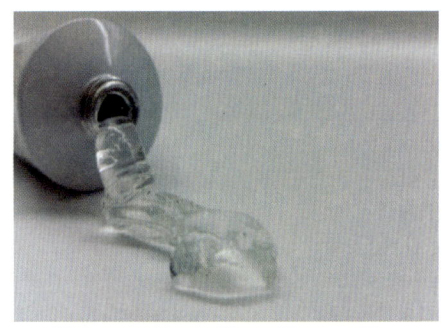

Paint

It is a viscous liquid preparation for application on skin or mucus membrane. They are made viscous so that the drug should remain in contact with mucous membrane for sufficiently longer time to produce its prolonged action.

Example: Gum paint

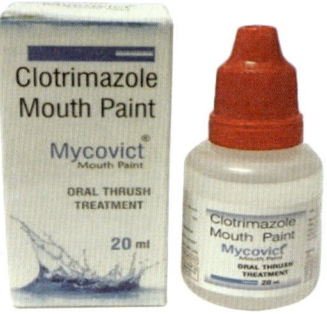

Spray

Sprays are aerosol preparations containing medicaments for topical application. Aerosols provide cooling effect and lesser irritation over abraded area. There is minimal wastage, no contamination of unused portion and faster absorption of the drug.

Example: Analgesic spray

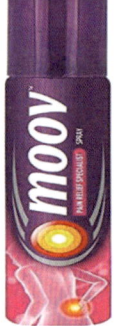

Enema

It is meant for rectal administration. It is employed to evacuate bowel (evacuation enema) or to produce local.

Example: Soap water enema. or systemic action (retention enema)

Example: Hydrocortisone rectal suspension.

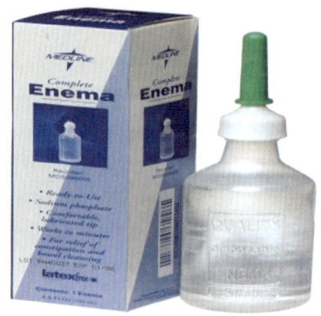

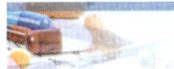

Mouthwash

It is an aqueous solution with a pleasant taste and colour used for rinsing, deodorant, refreshing or antiseptic action.
Example: Listerine, Colgate plax

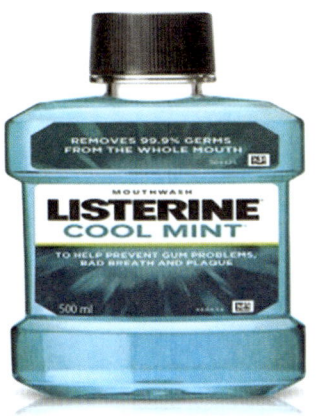

Irrigation solution

It is a sterile and pyrogen free solution of active ingredient in sterile water employed to wash or bathe surgical incisions, wounds or body cavities. For example, sodium chloride irrigation for washing wounds. Some irrigation solutions like douches, comes under this category they work as cleansing or antiseptic agents against a part or cavity of the body. They contain alum, zinc sulphate, boric acid, phenol or sodium borate.
Example: Vaginal douches.

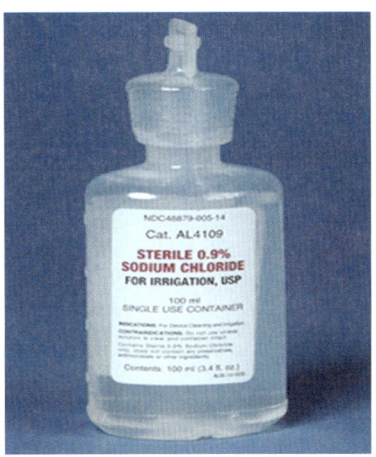

There are liquid preparation in the form of drops for topical use in eye, ear and nose externally. They are dispensed in plastic squeeze bottles or glass dropper bottles with a dropper cap usually with a capacity of 10–15 ml.

Eyedrops (Ophthalmic Solutions)

These are aqueous or oily solutions or suspensions of medicament, meant to be applied to conjunctiva, conjunctival sac or eyelids. For example, sulfacetamide eyedrops. Eye ointments have longer duration of action but eyes may become sticky due to greasy base. For example, chloramphenicol 1.0% w/w eye ointment, acyclovir eye ointment.

Method of Self Administration for Eye (Drops and Ointment)

1. Wash your hands.
2. Do not touch the dropper opening/tip of the tube.
3. Tilting head backward/laying down
4. Pulling lower eyelid using index finger for making eye 'gutter' or pocket
5. Apply/pour the prescribed amount of drop/ointment.
6. Close the eye for 2 min. after instilling the drop/ointment and do not shut the eye too tightly.
7. Excess fluid/ointment should be removed with the tissue paper.
8. If more than one kind of eyedrops is to be used wait at least 5 minutes before instilling the next drops.
9. Always check the label including expiry date.
10. Eyedrops may cause a burning feeling but this should not last for more than a few minutes. If it lasts longer consult the doctor.

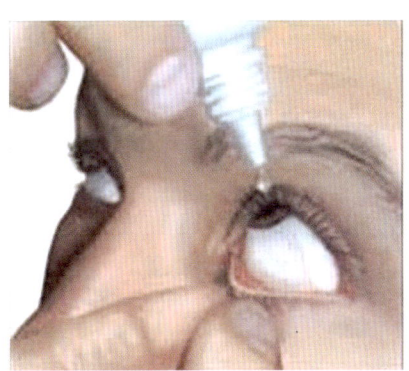

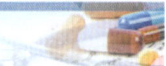

Eardrops

They are aqueous or viscous solutions of drugs to be instilled in external ear.

Example: Clotrimazole eardrops, ear wax removal drops.

Method of Instillation of Eardrops

1. Wash your hands.
2. Warm the eardrops by keeping them in the hand or the armpit for several minutes. Do not use hot water tap.
3. Tilt head sideways or lie on one side with the affected ear upward.
4. Gently pull the lobe to expose the ear canal.
5. Instill the amount of drops prescribed.
6. Wait for five minutes before turning to the other ear.
7. Use cotton wool to close the ear canal after applying the drops only if the manufacturer explicitly recommends this.

Nasal Spray

There are drugs or combinations of the drugs which by virtue of their high vapour pressure can be carried by an air current into nasal passage and exert their local and systemic effects. For example, Otrivin nasal spray (xylomethazoline hydrochloride). Nasal drops are another solutions of active ingredients in a vehicle suitable for instillation in the nose. They should not contain an oily base. Drops spread more extensively than the spray. For example, oxymethazoline hydrochloride nasal solution.

Method of instillation of nasal spray	Method of instillation of nasal drops
1. Blow the nose.	1. Blow the nose
2. *Sit with the head slightly tilted forward*	2. *Sit down and tilt head backwards or lie down with a pillow under the shoulders; keep head straight*
3. Shake the spray. Insert the tip in one nostril	3. Insert the dropper one centimeter into the nostril
4. Close the other nostril and mouth	4. Apply the amount of drops prescribed
5. Spray by squeezing the vial (flask, container) and sniff slowly	5. Immediately afterwards tilt head forward (head between knees)
6. Remove the tip from the nose and bend the head forward strongly (head between the knees)	6. Sit up after a few seconds. The drops will then drip into the pharynx
7. Sit up after few seconds; the spray will drip down the pharynx	7. Repeat the procedure for the other nostril, if necessary
8. Breathe through the mouth	8. Rinse the dropper with boiled water.
9. Repeat the procedure for the other nostril, if necessary	
10. Rinse the tip with the boiled water	

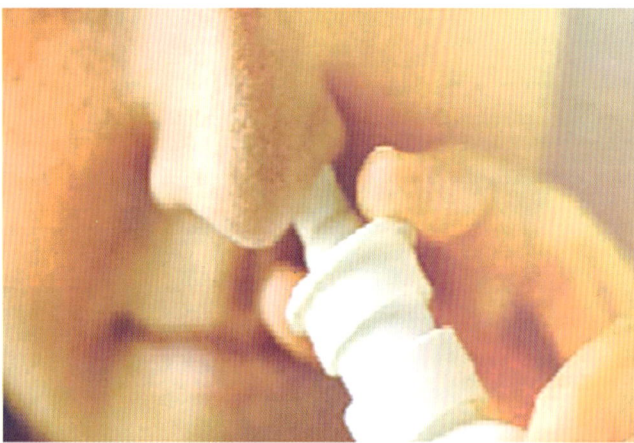

Head tilted forward (nasal spray)

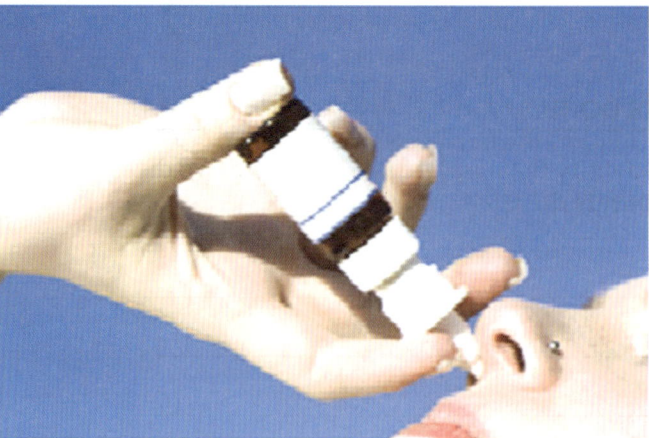

Head tilted brackward (nasal spray)

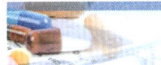

Liquid Parenteral Dosage forms

These are liquid preparations meant for parenteral administration. They must be sterile and pyrogen free.

Advantages of parenteral dosage forms

1. Faster action
2. Can be given in unconsciousness and uncooperative patients
3. Useful in patient with vomiting
4. First pass metabolism are avoided
5. Useful in emergency condition.

Disadvantages of parenteral dosages forms:

1. They required assistance and proper aseptic precautions
2. They may cause pain at injection site
3. They are expensive, inconvenient to patients
4. Injuries to nerve may occur.

Liquid dosage forms are available either in ampoule or vial.

1. **Ampoules:** It is a glass/plastic container, which contains single dose of a drug. The glass container has a neck portion which can be easily broken without fragmenting lower portion. Should be used immediately after broken.
   Example: Propofol, phenylephrine, etc.

2. **Multi-dose vial (bulb):** It contains multiple doses of drug solution or powder form of the drug. The solution can be reused but sterility has to be maintained. Vials have rubber or plastic cap which permits needle penetration and when needle is withdrawn the closure reseals and protects the solution from contaminants. When drug is in powdered form appropriate solvent is added in the recommended quantity to dissolve the drug. The unused drug should be preserved according to the manufacturer's instructions.
   Example: Hydromorphine hydrochloride injection.

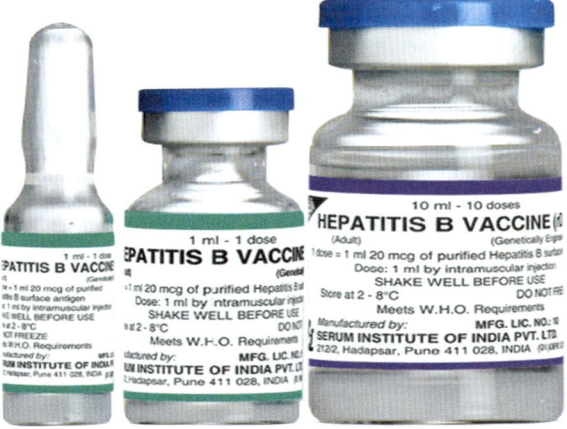

LET'S DO THIS

1. Identify the dosage form and write two disadvantages
   of this dosage form.

   _____

   _____

   _____

   _____

   _____

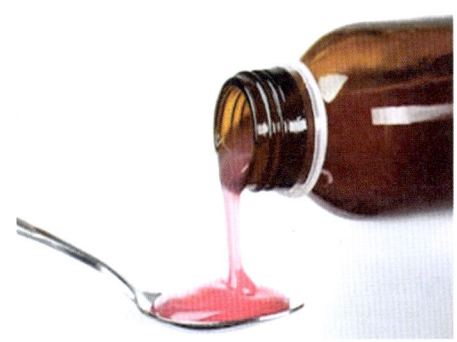

2. Write difference between vial and ampoule.

_____

_____

_____

_____

_____

3. What is draught?

_____

_____

_____

_____

_____

4. Identify the dosage form and write two advantages of this dosage form.

_____

_____

_____

_____

_____

_____

_____

_____

5. What should be the position of head in case of nasal spray and nasal drops instillation?

_____

_____

_____

_____

_____

6. True/False:
   i. Solutions are meant for internal use only _____
   ii. Emulsions are mixture of two immiscible solids. _____
   iii. Head should be tilted forward during nasal spray instillation
                                                              _____
   iv. Ampoule is also known as bulb _____

7. Instill 1 eyedrop in right eye in a given simulator. (Assessment by checklist of steps)

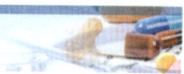

Date:

PRACTICAL 4

COMPETENCY

PH 2.1: Demonstrate understanding of the use of various dosage forms (oral/local/parenteral; solid/liquid)
PH 1.3: Enumerate and identify drug formulations and drug delivery system

Objectives

At the end of the practical class the student should be able to:
- Identify and list the common inhalational dosage forms.
- Enlist advantage and disadvantages of inhalational dosage forms.
- Demonstrate steps of meter dose inhaler with or without spacer in simulator environment.
- Demonstrate steps of nebulizer in simulator environment.

Domain: Knowledge and communication
Level: Shows how
Teaching learning methods: Small group discussion, DOAP
Aligning assessment methods: Skill assessment, OSPE with checklist, viva voce
Number of procedure to be done independently for certification: None

Materials Needed

Sample of meter dose inhaler, spacer, rotahaler, nebulizer and drugs, etc.

Inhalational dosage forms are aerosols containing drug particles or solutions to be administer by respiratory route for the treatment of respiratory disease like asthma, rhinitis. For example, salbutamol, terbutaline, etc. Liquid gas propellants are used to supply necessary force to expel the drug and also act as solvent and diluents. For inhalations, maximum size of dispersible particles of 5–10 µm may be used.

Advantages of inhalational dosage forms
- Rapid absorption due to large surface area
- Targeted higher concentration of drug delivery
- Rapid onset of action
- Less systemic side effects.

Disadvantages of inhalational dosage forms
- Irritant to bronchial mucosa
- May be costly
- Special techniques need to know.

It can be administered by
- Pressurised aerosol systems (metered dose inhaler with or without spacer)
- Dry powder systems (rotahaler)
- Nebuliser.

1. Metered Dose Inhaler (MDI)

They are compact, portable self-contained units that deliver fixed quantity of drug when a button on the top of the device is pressed. Pressurized aerosols produce fine mists. Good coordination is required to synchronize deep inspiration with release of drug. They are more cost effective than dry powder inhaler. High pharyngeal deposition of particle and difficult to determine remaining doses are the main drawback. Nowadays advanced MDI displaying remaining numbers of doses after each dose are available.

Steps of using meter dose inhaler

1. Take out the cap and clean the mouthpiece
2. Shake the inhaler before use
3. Exhale completely
4. Place the mouthpiece between lips

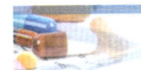

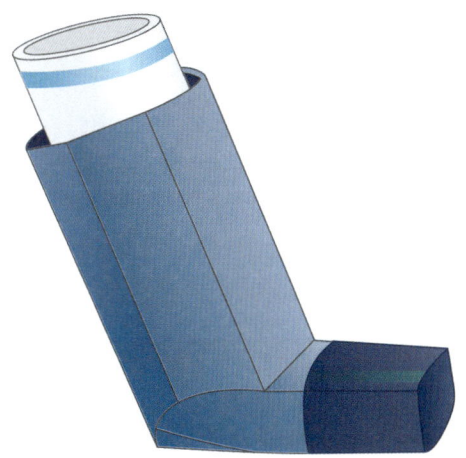

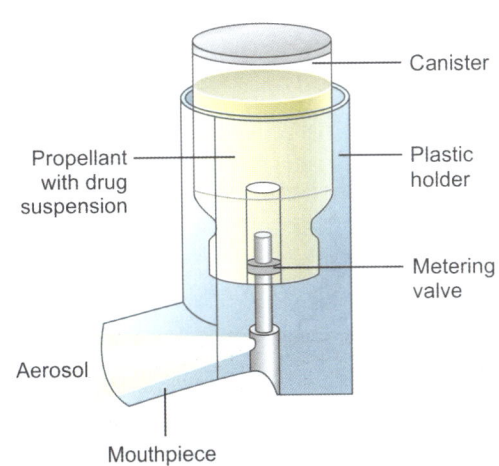

5. Tilt the head backward and press the inhaler while inhaling slowly and deeply
6. Hold breath in inspiration for 10 seconds at least or as long as comfortable
7. Wait for at least one minute before puffing the next dose
8. Gargles

2. Metered Dose Inhaler with Spacer

Spacer is a device which can be attached to an inhaler. This modification is made to overcome some drawbacks of metered dose inhaler. It can be used in children, elderly and addition of mask allows its use in infants also. Drug is released into a chamber/spacer from which the patient can inhale. Hence strict synchronization is not required between release of drug and inhalation. Deposition of drug in posterior pharynx is less as compared to metered dose inhaler and there is no wastage of drug. It is effective even when ventilation is impaired but it is less portable.

Steps of using meter dose inhaler with spacer

1. Prepare the spacer
2. Take out the cap of inhaler
3. Hold the inhaler upright and shake well and insert into spacer
4. Put mouthpiece between teeth and close lips to seal mouthpiece
5. Breathe out gently into spacer
6. Hold spacer level and press down firmly on canister
7. Single breath
8. Breath out gently
9. Remove inhaler from spacer
10. Gargles

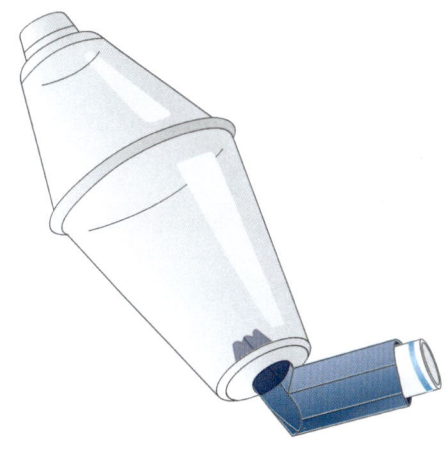

3. Dry Powder Inhaler

Dry powder inhalers are portable devices suitable for patients who have difficulty with MDIs and do not require coordination with inspiration while using it. These are breath activated, i.e. drug is released only when person takes a deep and fast breath in through the inhaler. Inspiratory flow rates govern the amount of drug delivered which may vary in individuals with lung disorders. Micronized drug particles (2–5 µm) are mixed with carrier particles to make a free flowing powder. When inhaled the turbulence created by inhaler and the energy of inspired air flow liberate drug particles (which reach lungs) from the surface of carrier particles (which deposit on the oropharynx and swallowed).

They might be pre-metered or device metered available in many different designs. The pre-metered inhalers contain fix doses in form of capsules, blisters, etc. which are either inserted into the device during manufacturing or by the patient before use. Device metered inhalers have an internal reservoir of multiple doses that are metered by the device itself. For example, spinhaler/rotahaler in which the drug is supplied as a powder in a capsule. Two small pins are provided in a spin inhaler. When required the pin pierces the capsule to release the drug and the drug blows out as the patient inhales.

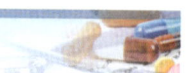

Steps of using rotahaler

1. Insert rota capsule's transparent end into square hole
2. Press rota capsule firmly
3. Hold the mouthpiece firmly with one hand and rotate the base with another hand
4. Exhale completely
5. Place the mouthpiece between teeth and seal with lips
6. Inhaling completely through the mouth
7. Hold the breath as long as possible
8. Gargles.

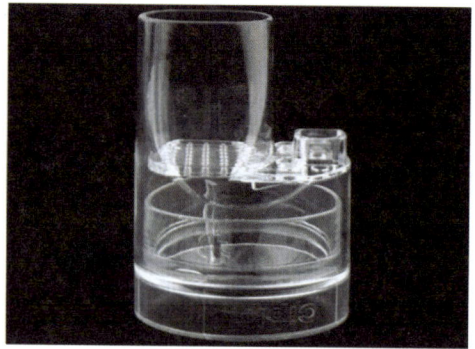
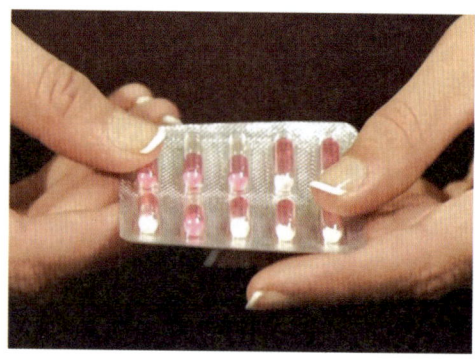

4. Nebuliser

Nebulizer is a bigger device used for inhalation of drug solutions especially during emergency. It generates fine droplets of uniform size which reach the bronchioles. It is effective even when ventilation is impaired. Dose of the drug delivered is much larger than metered dose inhaler. It is less portable and there may be chances of over dosage.

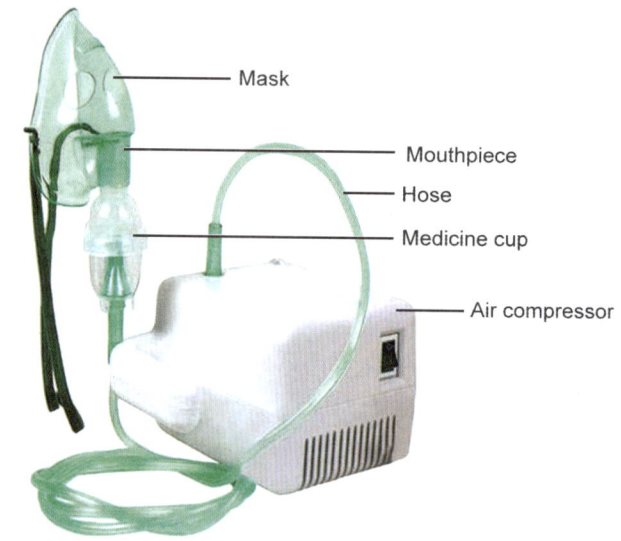

Steps of administration of nebulizer

1. Assemble the nebulizer according to instructions given on the manual of the nebulizer. Connect the tube/hose to an air compressor
2. Fill the nebulizer/medicine cup with the drug solution prescribed
3. Attach the hose and mouthpiece to the medicine cup
4. Place the mouthpiece in the mouth and ask the patient to breath until all the medicine is used up (around 10–15 min). Nose clip can be used to help to breathe only through mouth
5. Wash the medicine cup after each use.

LET'S DO THIS

1. a. Identify the device.
   b. What are disadvantages of it over MDI?

   _____

   _____

   _____

   _____

   _____

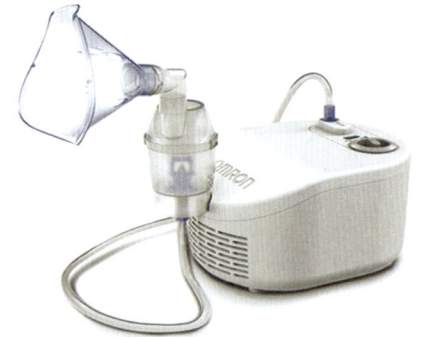

2. a. Write the name of this device used with MDI.
   b. Write its advantages.

_____

_____

_____

_____

_____

_____

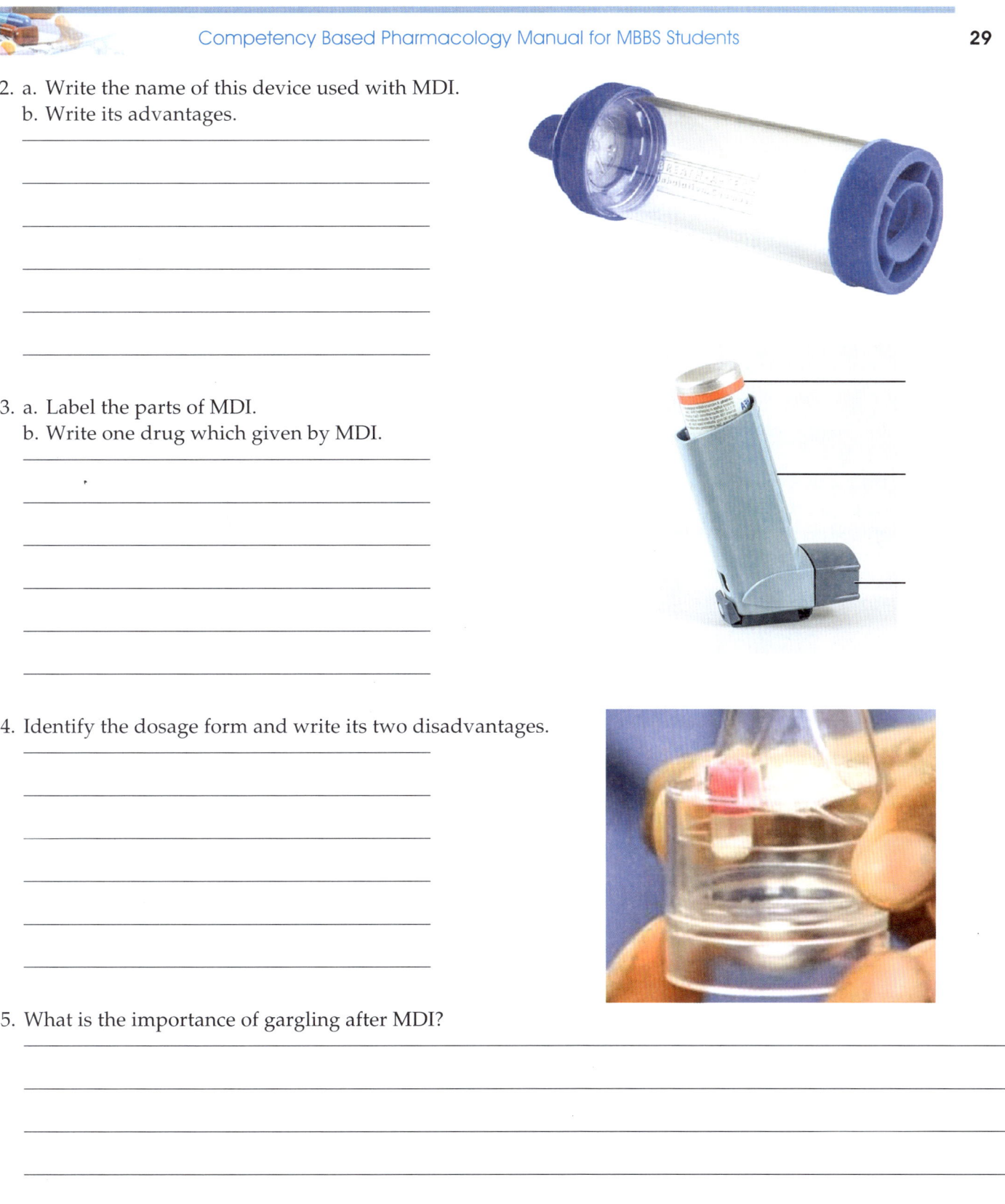

3. a. Label the parts of MDI.
   b. Write one drug which given by MDI.

_____

_____

_____

_____

_____

_____

4. Identify the dosage form and write its two disadvantages.

_____

_____

_____

_____

_____

5. What is the importance of gargling after MDI?

_____

_____

_____

_____

_____

_____

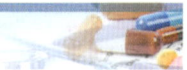

Date:

PRACTICAL 5

COMPETENCY

PH2.1: Demonstrate understanding of the use of various dosage forms (oral/local/parenteral; solid/liquid)
PH1.3: Enumerate and identify drug formulations and drug delivery system

Objectives

At the end of the practical class the student should be able to:
• Identify the special drug delivery system.
• Enlist advantage and disadvantages of special drug delivery system.

Domain: Knowledge and communication
Level: Shows how
Teaching learning methods: Small group discussion, DOAP
Aligning assessment methods: Skill assessment, viva voce
Number of procedure to be done independently for certification: None

Materials Needed

Sample of various special drug delivery system like transdermal patch, insulin pen, etc.

Newer drug delivery systems have been developed to overcome the limitations of the conventional drug delivery systems. There are various advantages of this delivery system except that they are mostly costly.

Advantages of Special Drug Delivery Systems

• Increased drug potency
• Increased efficacy of the drug
• Decreased toxicity/side effects
• Maintain steady state plasma concentration
• Increased patient compliance
• Viable treatment for previously incurable disease.

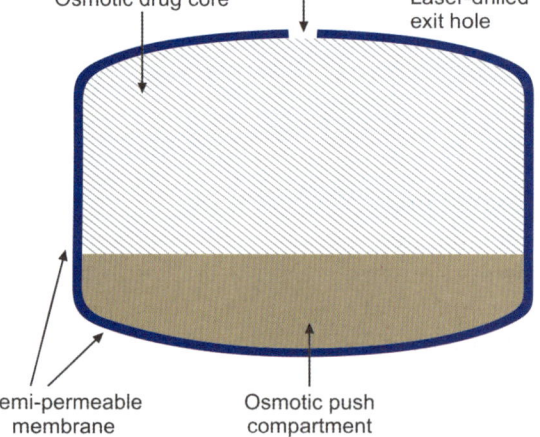

1. Modified Oral Drug Delivery System

Few modifications in tablets like enteric coated, sustained release tablet and spansules which make them gastro resistant and longer acting; already been explained in oral solid dosage forms.

Prodrugs

These are designed as pharmacologically inactive forms and get activated in the body by biotransformation. Prodrugs may be used to prolong the duration action of drug like Bacampicillin (Prodrug of ampicillin) and also to increase the concentration of at particular site like Levodopa (Prodrug of Dopamine) which is used to treat parkinsonism because dopamine cannot cross the blood–brain barrier.

Osmotic pumps

They consist of a drug core containing osmogen (osmotically active) that is coated with a semi permeable membrane. This coating has one or more orifice on coating through which a solution or suspension of the drug after ingestion of water, is pumped out osmotically over a period of time.
Example: Nifedipine, glipizide in osmotic formulation, etc.

2. Polymer Based Delivery System

These are drug delivery devices made of polymers which have to be implanted subcutaneously or in various body cavities requiring surgical intervention. They are useful for chronic administration of drugs as the drug is released in controlled manner.

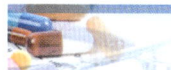

Progestasert
It is the intrauterine device used for contraception which consists of drug saturated liquid medium encapsulated in a polymeric membrane. It releases progesterone at constant rate for a period of one year.

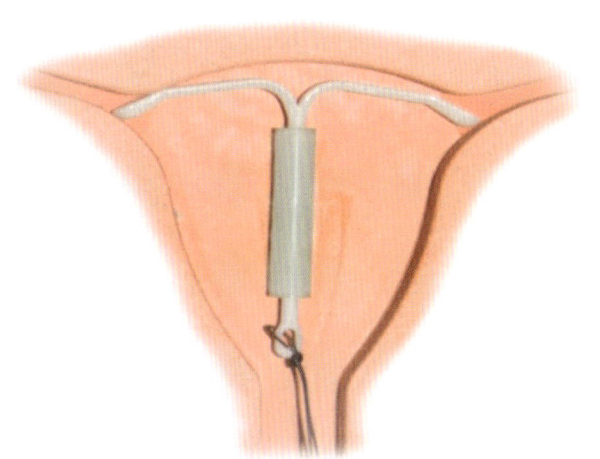

Ocusert or Ocular insert
It is a novel means of controlled ocular drug delivery in which is a thin elliptical device containing drug is placed in the eye just like contact lens.
Example: Pilocarpine ocusert. Inserted in cul-de-sac, lachrymal fluid enters the system and the dissolved drug slowly gets released through polymeric membrane.

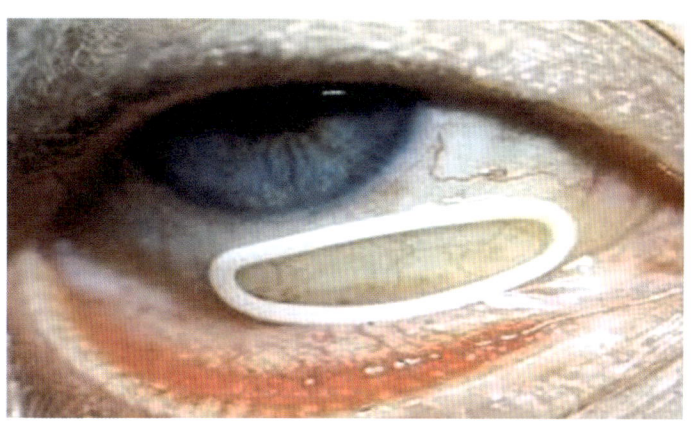

Coated implantable devices
Metallic stent covered with polymer containing drugs known as drugs eluting stunts.
Example: Sirolimus or Paclitaxel. Drugs slowly release over 2–4 weeks.

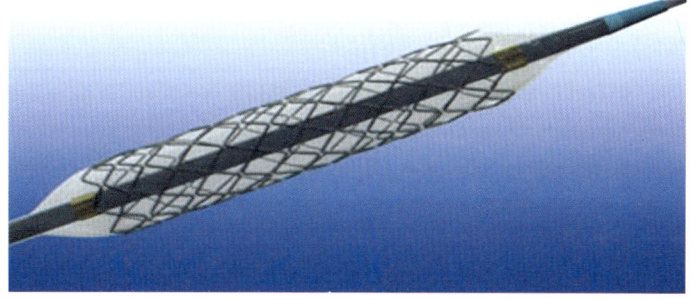

3. Transdermal Drug Delivery Systems

These are adhesive patches or discs of various sizes that may be attached to the body permitting controlled release of drugs via stratum corneum. Drugs held in reservoir between occlusive backing film and rate controlling micropore membrane smeared with adhesive impregnated with priming dose of drugs—covered with protective layer. The pores of the membrane are filled with a fluid, which is highly permeable to the drug. Protective layer should be removed before application to enable the drug release. An adhesive layer in the system helps to maintain contact with the skin after application. This delivery system increase duration of action and provide constant plasma levels of drugs. Most common sites for application are chest, abdomen, upper arm, lower back, buttock and mastoid region. For example, clonidine, glyceryl trinitrate, nicotine, etc.

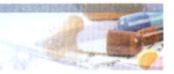

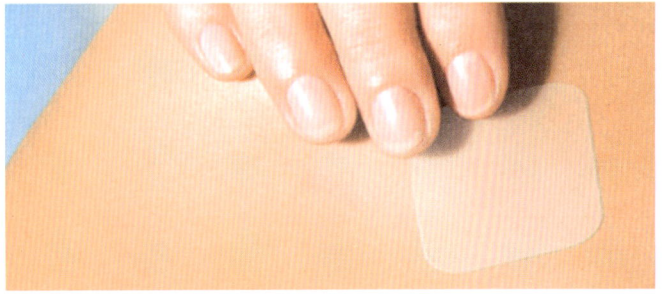

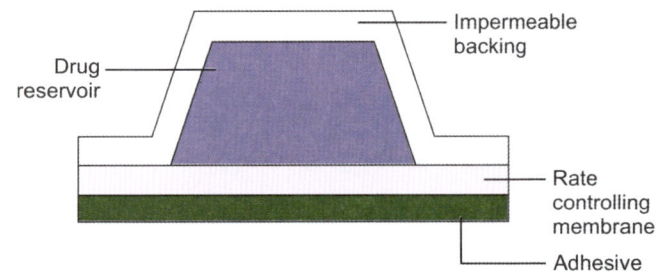

4. Carrier Based Targeted Drug Delivery Systems

In this system drug delivery is possible only by means of a carrier molecule and various methods of drug targeting (to deliver drug at the site) are used mainly for anticancer drugs to decreases adverse effects and toxicities.

Liposome

Liposomes are the vesicles composed of an aqueous core bounded by a hydrophobic lipid bilayer. These liposomes can be used as carriers for both water and lipid soluble drugs since they can be trapped in the aqueous spaces or within lipid bilayers respectively. They can be used to deliver drugs to blood, bone marrow, liver, spleen and lymphoid organs. Their plasma half-life ranges from minutes to several hours. For example, Amphotericin B, Doxorubicin, Daunorubicin.

Polymer-drug conjugates

Polymer-drug conjugates comprise of water soluble polymer being conjugated to a drug chemically with the help of a biodegradable coupler. For example, PEG-interferon α, PEG-adenosine deaminase, etc.

Monoclonal antibodies

The antibodies synthesized against a particular antigen are known as monoclonal antibodies. They are so called because they arise from a single cell type. Monoclonal antibodies are a class of highly specific antibodies produced by the clones of a single hybrid cell formed in the laboratory by the fusion of B-lymphocytes with a specific cell. Because of their high specificity they can be used as targeted delivery system for destroying diseased tissue only. For example, trastuzumab, rituximab.

Nanotechnology

Drug delivery at nanoscale has become possible due to the development and fabrication of nanostructures. Nanotechnology is popularly known as science of small or scientifically described as the technology to develop materials and structures of the size range from 1 to 100 nanometers; which can be used as carriers for drugs. These carriers are negatively charged sphericals with amorphous and lipophilic surfaces. There sizes can vary between 10 nm and 1000 nm depending on manufacturing process and pores vary between 3 nm and 6 nm. They are administered parenterally. For example, gold nanoparticles in treatment of breast, prostate cancer.

5. Newer Insulin Drug Delivery System

Insulin is given as subcutaneous injection in patients of Type I diabetes mellitus for lifelong period. Various newer drug delivery systems have been developed for delivering insulin to increase the patient's compliance.

Insulin Pen device

These are like ordinary writing pen with an insulin cartridge inside. At one end specially designed replaceable needle is attached to cartridge. A fixed dose of insulin can be given with the help of a dial which can be set according to dose required. A push button of plunger emerges as the dose is dialled and insulin is delivered when it is pressed.

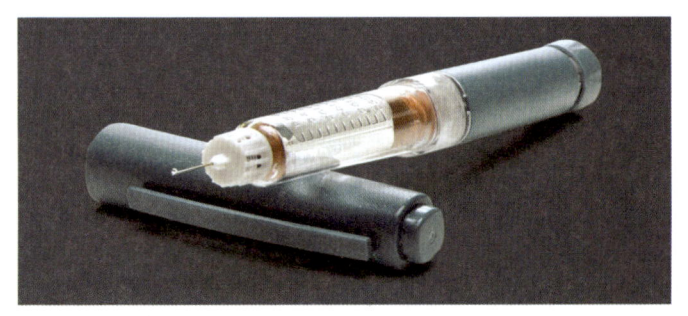

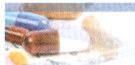

Jet injector

Jet injector forces insulin under high pressure through nozzle. Microjet stream penetrates the skin and disperses subcutaneously.

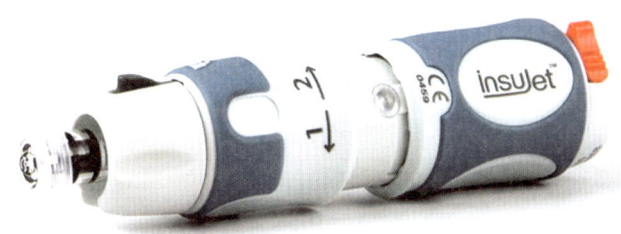

Continuous subcutaneous Infusion (CSII) pumps

Portable continuous infusion pumps are an external open loop pump with a size of a pager which can be placed on belt or pocket. The use is encouraged for individuals who are unable to obtain target control while on multiple injection regimens. Chances of infection are main drawback.

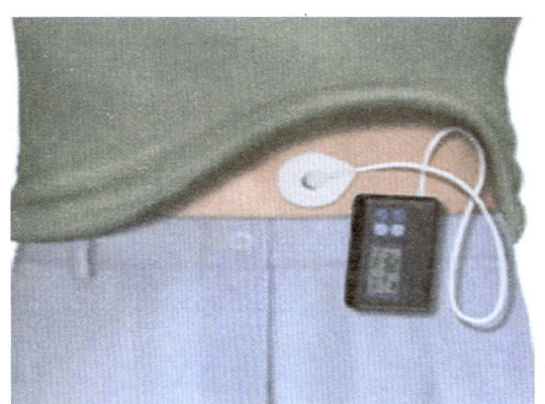

Inhaled insulin

Inhalers containing rDNA human insulin in powdered or aerosolized form are delivered through a nebulizer.
Example: Alfrezza

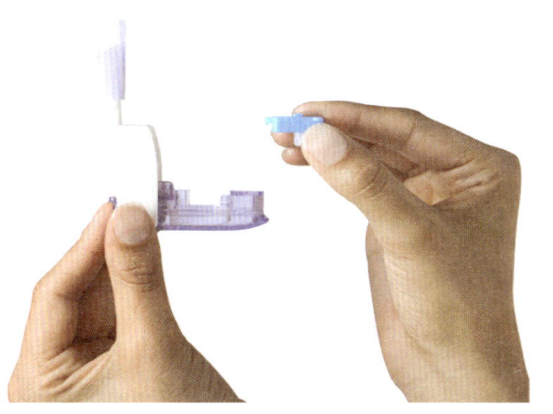

LET'S DO THIS

1. a. Identify the type of drug delivery system.
   b. Write two drugs given by this system.

   _____

   _____

   _____

   _____

   _____

   _____

   _____

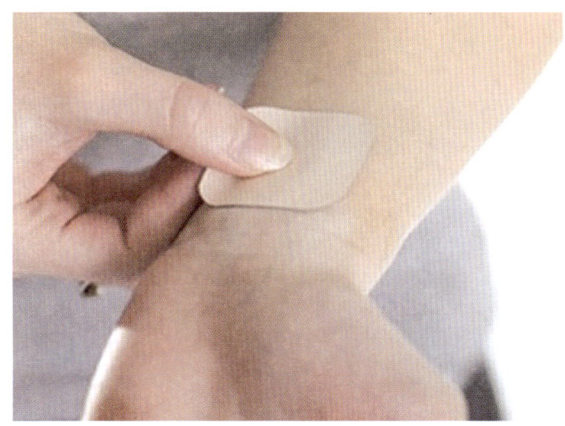

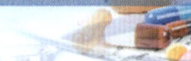

2. a. Identify the instrument.
   b. Write one drug given by this device.

   _____

   _____

   _____

   _____

   _____

   _____

   _____

3. Write advantages of ocusert drug delivery system.

   _____

   _____

   _____

   _____

   _____

   _____

4. Write two carrier molecules which are used in targeted drug delivery systems.

   _____

   _____

   _____

   _____

   _____

   _____

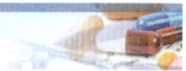

Date:

PRACTICAL 6

COMPETENCY PH2.2

Prepare oral rehydration solution from ORS packet and explain its use.

Objectives

At the end of this practical class, student should be able to:

- Explain steps for preparation of ORS solution
- List advantages and disadvantage of ORS
- Explain the rationale of ORS in diarrhoea
- Prescribe and dispense ORS.

Domain: Skill and communication
Level: Shows how
Teaching learning methods: Small group discussion, DOAP, role play
Aligning assessment methods: Skill Assessment, OSPE with checklist, viva voce
Number of procedure to be done independently for certification: None

Material Needed

ORS powder, distilled water, beaker (container), simulated patient.

According to World Health Organization (WHO), diarrhoea is defined as passage of three or more loose or liquid stools per day or more frequent passage than is normal for an individual. Depending upon the duration; diarrhoea can be acute, persistent or chronic. Massive diarrhoea with watery stools may result in a marked depletion of sodium, potassium, and bicarbonates and ultimately metabolic acidosis. Hence, replacement of fluid and electrolyte loss forms the most important therapeutic aspect of dehydration. There are two types of rehydration depending upon severity of dehydration: Intravenous and Oral rehydration.

Rationale of ORS composition

- Oral Rehydration Salt/Solution/Therapy (ORS/ORT) is designed to maintain and restore hydration, electrolyte and pH balance until diarrhoea ceases or within 6 hours.
- Recommended for mild (5–7% body weight) or moderate (7–10% body weight) fluid loss.
- Initially, ORS formula contained sodium bicarbonate along with Na^+, K^+, Cl^- and glucose.
- In 1984, WHO recommended formula containing trisodium citrate instead of sodium bicarbonate because bicarbonate containing ORS powder had a shorter shelf-life and developed brown colour due to furfural compound formation with glucose.
- K^+ is important as lost in diarrhoea. Citrate corrects acidosis due to alkali loss in stools and promotes Na^+ and water absorption. Glucose is indicated to help the absorption of Na^+ and not as a source of energy.
- However, this old ORS formula caused periorbital oedema due to excess Na^+ absorption from intestine.
- This led to new modified WHO-ORS formula in 2002.

Table 6.1: Old WHO-ORS formula			
Substance	**Weight**	**Components**	**mmol/litre**
Sodium chloride	3.5 g	Na^+	90
Potassium chloride	1.5 g	K^+	20
Trisodium citrate	2.9 g	Citrate	10
Glucose	20 g	Chloride	80
Water	1 L	Glucose	111
		Total osmolarity	311

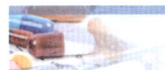

Table 6.2: New modified WHO-ORS formula			
Substance	**Weight**	**Components**	**mmol/litre**
Sodium chloride	2.6 g	Na^+	75
Potassium chloride	1.5 g	K^+	20
Trisodium citrate	2.9 g	Citrate	10
Glucose	13.5 g	Chloride	65
Water	1 L	Glucose	75
		Total osmolarity	245

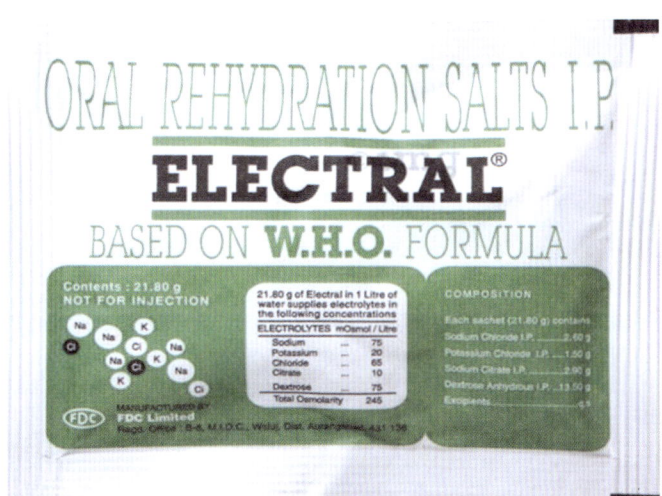

Advantages of ORS

- Easy, simple, less expensive and an effective therapy.
- Reduces stool volume by 20% and vomiting by 30%.
- Faster water absorption.
- Low risk of hypernatremia.
- Effective and safe in cholera too.
- Potassium replacement is safer orally than intravenous.
- No risk of fluid overload, pulmonary congestion and oedema.
- Effective for all age groups.
- No expertise is needed, can be administered at home.

Disadvantages of ORS

It is difficult to administer in presence of vomiting or shock.

Steps for Preparation of ORS Solution

- Wash hands with soap and water before preparing ORS.
- Pour 1 litre of drinking water in a container.
- Empty the contents of ORS sachet into the container (1 litre water) and stir until contents dissolve completely.
- Administer ORS as much as per the patient's requirements and degree of dehydration at regular intervals.
- Do not store it after 24 hours and discard the leftover.

Administration of ORS

- **Treatment plan A:** Treatment of diarrhoea in children with NO dehydration. If the child is less than 2 years old, teaspoonful should be given every 1–2 minutes. For an older child, frequent sips from a cup can be given. If the child vomits it out, wait for 10 minutes. Later give the solution more slowly, i.e. every 2–3 minutes.

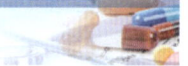

Table 6.3: Treatment Plan A of ORS	
Age	**Amount of ORS** **(Given after every loose stool)**
<24 months	50–100 ml/loose stool
2–10 years	100–200 ml/loose stool
10 years or above	As much as child wants
If ORS not available, homemade available fluid can be used	

- **Treatment plan B:** Treatment of diarrhoea in children with some dehydration. Commencement of ORS for the correction of existing water and electrolyte loss as well as maintenance of normal daily fluid requirements.
- **Treatment plan C:** Treatment of diarrhoea in children with severe dehydration [severe fluid loss, i.e. >10% body weight or >10 ml/kg/hr or unable to tolerate ORS (weakness, vomiting)]. For intravenous rehydration, Dhaka fluid or Ringer Lactate is administered. Volume equivalent to 10% body weight should be infused over 2–4 hours and later shifted to oral rehydration.

Other Types of ORS

- Super ORS = Adding of Glycine (amino acid) results in improvements in sodium and water absorption but very expensive.
- Rice water ORS = Glucose 20 gm is replaced by 50 gm of cooked rice powder, provides more calories.
- Wheat, mazie, potato or cereal based ORS.

Home-made Fluids

- Rice water, lemon juice, fruit juices, coconut water, tea and coffee, buttermilk, soups.
- (Lemon juice = Fist of sugar (20 g) + 1 pinch of salt (5 g) + ½ lemon + 1 litre of water).

Zinc in Pediatric Diarrhoea

- Addition of zinc reduces the duration and severity of acute diarrhoea in children less than 5 years age by reducing the fluid loss, strengthening immunity and regenerating intestinal epithelium.
- WHO, UNICEF and IAP recommends zinc supplementation to all children with acute diarrhoea for 10–14 days with a dose of 10 mg/day (<6 months age) and 20 mg/day (children and adults).

Non-diarrhoeal Uses of ORS/ORT

- Post-surgical, post-burn and post-trauma maintenance of hydration and nutrition.
- Heat stroke.
- During change over from intravenous to enteral alimentation.

LET'S DO THIS

1. Why glucose is added in ORS?

_____

_____

_____

_____

2. Write two home-made fluids.

_____

_____

_____

3. Why trisodium citrate was added in WHO ORS instead of sodium bicarbonate?

_____

_____

_____

_____

_____

_____

4. What do you mean by compound powder? Is ORS a simple or compound powder?

_____

_____

_____

_____

_____

_____

_____

5. Write two advantages of ORS.

_____

_____

_____

_____

_____

6. Perform role play in simulated environment regarding communication to the mother of child less than 2 years of age about ORS use. Few students will observe and comments on the activity done. At the end teacher with give his/her suggestion to improve upon.

_____

_____

_____

_____

_____

_____

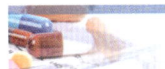

Date:

PRACTICAL 7

COMPETENCY PH2.3

Demonstrate the appropriate setting up of an intravenous drip in a simulated environment

Objectives

At the end of this practical class student should be able to:

- Enlist advantages and disadvantages of IV infusion
- Demonstrate the parts of IV set
- Set up an IV drip in a simulated environment
- Calculate the flow rate and total time of infusion for a given clinical situation.

Domain: Skill
Level: Shows how
Teaching learning methods: Small group discussion, DOAP
Aligning assessment methods: Skill assessment, OSPE with checklist, viva voce
Number of procedure to be done independently for certification: None

Material Needed

Drugs, needle, syringe, spirit swab, IV cannula, fixing tape, IV fluid, IV set, IV injection arm (mannequin), IV stand, gloves

Indications for Intravenous (IV) Infusion

- To administer fluid in case hypovolemia/dehydration, shock, burn, perioperative period, etc.
- Medications such as potassium chloride, heparin, lignocaine, quinine and most antibiotics, corticosteroids, vitamins are best given intermittently with IV infusion set.
- To maintain constant plasma level of the drug. For example, norepinepherine, insulin, dopamine.
- When it is necessary to control/titrate the dose according to the need. For example, NTG, sodium nitroprusside for emergency control of hypertension.
- For total parenteral nutrition (TPN).

Intravenous Fluids

Parenteral fluid therapy involves the intravenous administration of crystalloid solutions, colloidal solutions and/or blood products. These are most commonly used to provide water, electrolytes, and nutrients to meet daily requirements and also to administer medications and blood products through IV infusion. They are available in glass or plastic containers in 100 ml, 500 ml or 1000 ml capacity. For example, normal saline 0.9%, 3%, dextrose solutions 5%, 10%, 20%, 25%, dextrose normal saline, Ringer's lactate, Ringer acetate, isolyte P

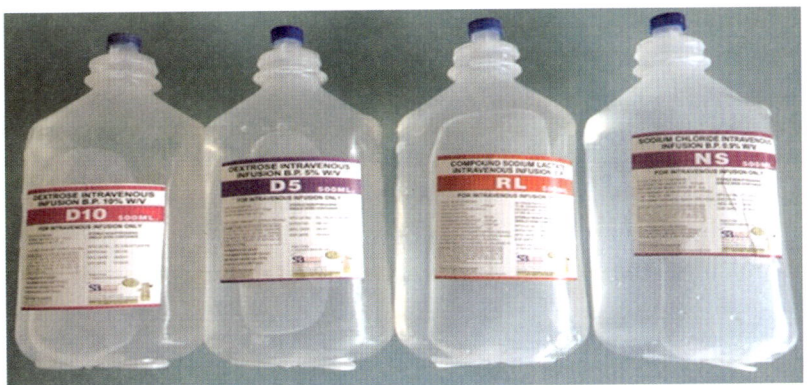

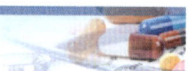

Problems Associated with IV Infusion

- Thrombophlebitis of injected vein.
- Necrosis of adjoining tissues on extravasation.
- Sloughing on injection of irritating substances.
- Infection.
- No retreat once the drug is injected.

Parts of IV Set

Spike (plunger) = for fixing into the IV fluid bottle
Drip chamber (Murphy's chamber) = with filter (for blood transfusion) or without filter to fix the drop rate.
Plastic tubing = for passage of fluids.
Control clamp (or roller or regulator) = to control rate of flow.
Latex tube = for injecting additional drugs.
Needle adapter = to be introduced inside the needle.

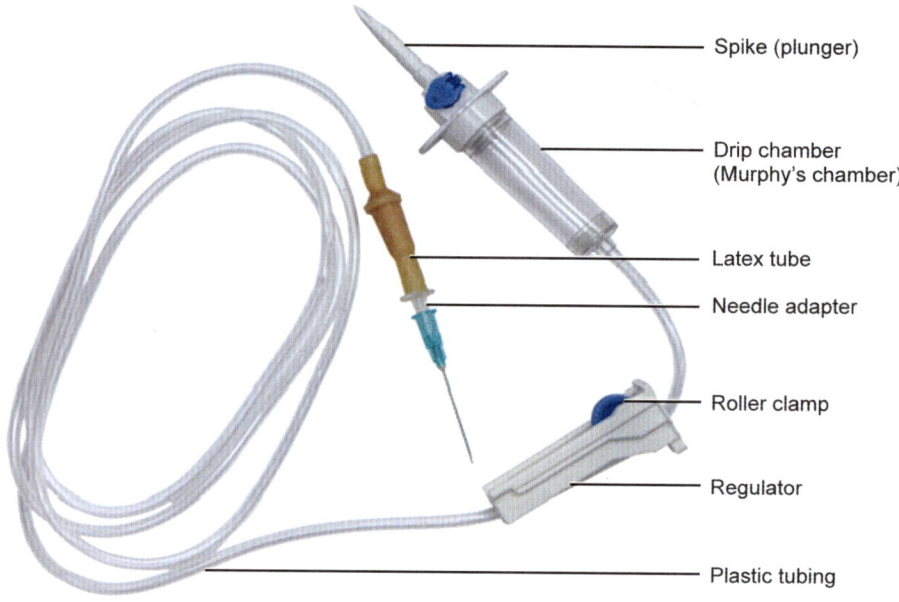

Spike (plunger)

Drip chamber
(Murphy's chamber)

Latex tube

Needle adapter

Roller clamp

Regulator

Plastic tubing

Parts of infusion set

Procedure for Setting up an IV Infusion

1. Observe aseptic precaution.
2. Reassure and explain the procedure to patient.
3. Remove the bottle from plastic bag. Remove the nipple-cap from the bottle in case of a plastic bottle and remove the sheet cover off the cork in case of a glass bottle.
4. Take out the IV set from the plastic bag
5. Attach needle to the adapter of the IV set.
6. Close the roller-clamp (regulator) by bringing the wheel at the bottom of the roller-clamp.
7. Insert the spike of the set into the bottle by giving 2–3 clockwise jerks.
8. Turn the bottle upside down and hang it at a suitable length. Insert the air vent, if needed.
9. Squeeze and release the drip-chamber until it is half filled.
10. Open the roller-clamp and allow the solution to run a little. This ensures the removal of the air from the IV set. Now close the roller-clamp.

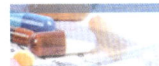

11. Apply the spirit swab over the exposed skin, perform the venepuncture using a sterile IV cannula and fix it using fixing tape. (Separate competency discussed with routes)
12. Open the roller-clamp and adjust the flow rate.

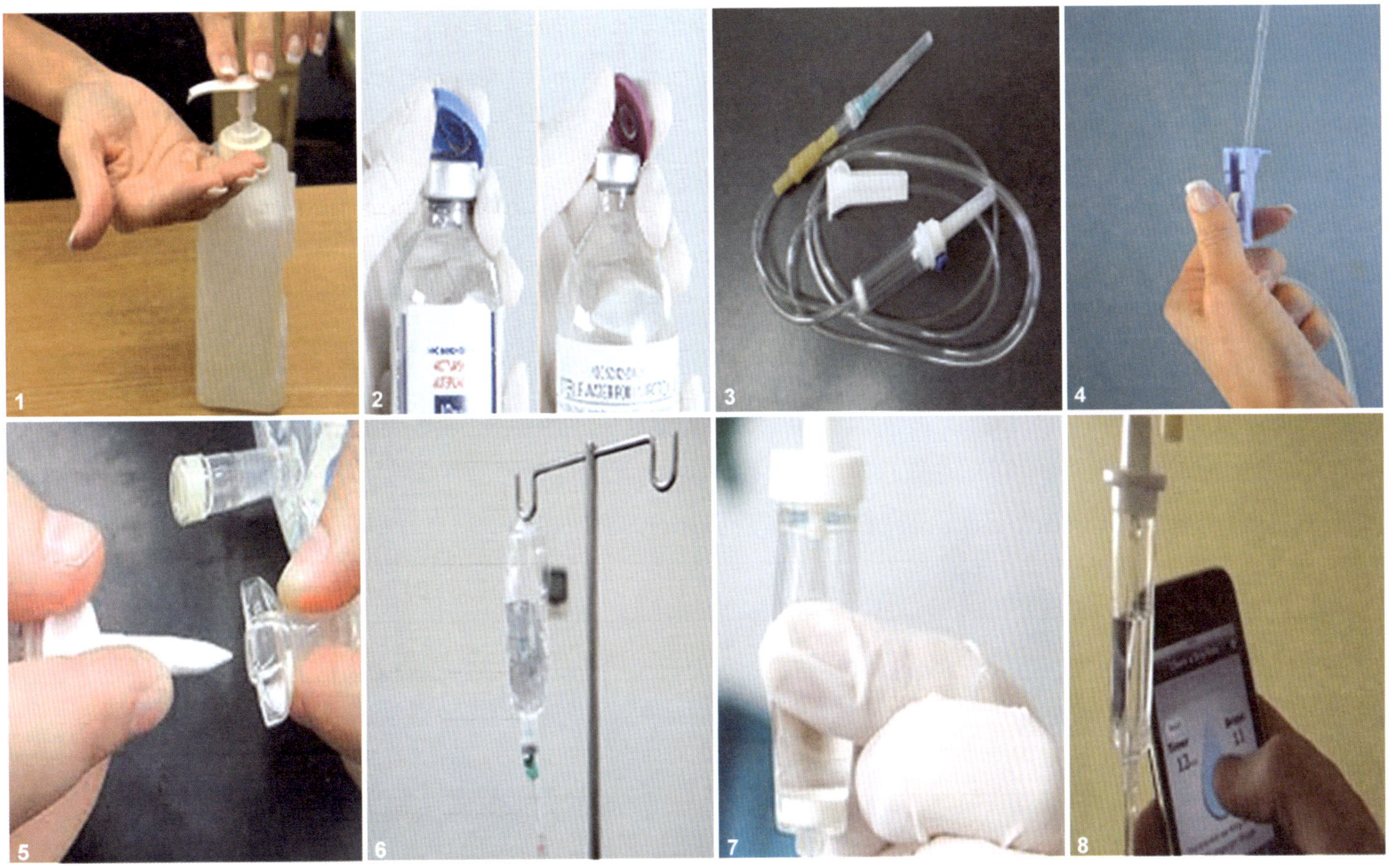

Calculation Example

Calculate the infusion rate (drops/min) and the time (in hrs) required to administer the infusion of dopamine in 500 ml of 5% dextrose solution for an adult patient weighing 80 kg. Dose required is 2 mcg/kg/min. One ampoule of dopamine contains 200 mg/5 ml. (1 ml of dopamine is added in 500 ml of dextrose)

Weight of patient = 80 kg

Dose = 2 mcg/kg/min

Therefore, dose required for the patient = 2 × 80 = 160 mcg/min

5 ml of dopamine vial contains = 200 mg

So, 1 ml contains = 40 mg

This 1 ml of dopamine is added in 500 ml of dextrose

So, the strength of solution is 40 × 1000 mcg/500 = 80 mcg/ml (1 mg = 1000 mcg)

Now, requirement of patient = 160 mcg/min

Therefore, 2ml/min should be infused to administer a dose of 2 mcg/kg/min.

If 1 ml = 16 drops, we will have to infuse 32 drops/min.

As 2 ml take 1 min, and 500 ml bottle to be infused

Total time required for infusion will be 500/2 = 250 minutes (~4 hours 10 minutes).

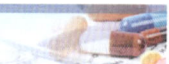

Let's do this:

1. Label the parts of IV set.

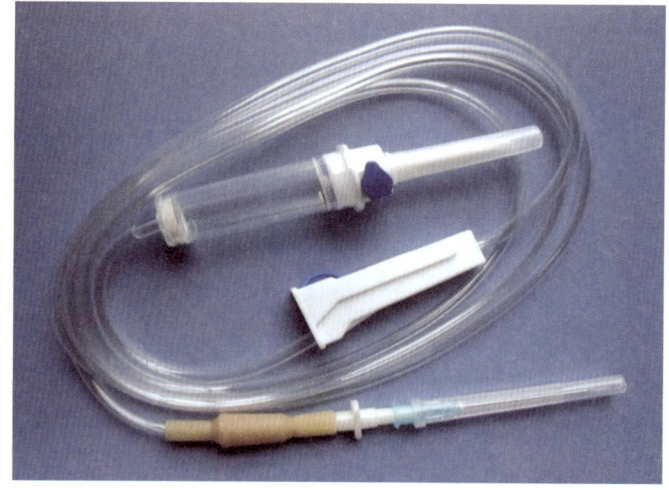

2. Why filter is present in drip chamber of blood transfusion set?

_____

_____

_____

_____

_____

_____

_____

_____

_____

_____

3. Which types of drugs are given by IV infusion? Write one example.

_____

_____

_____

_____

_____

_____

_____

_____

_____

_____

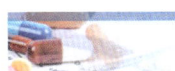

4. Find out the infusion rate (drops/min) and the time required (in hrs) to administer the infusion of dobutamine in 500 ml of 5% dextrose solution for an adult patient (55 yr, wt. 60 kg) at the rate of 5 mcg/kg/min. One ampoule of 5 ml contains 250 mg of dobutamine.

_____

_____

_____

_____

_____

_____

_____

_____

_____

_____

_____

_____

_____

5. Find out the infusion rate (drops/min) and the time required (in hrs) to administer the infusion of aminophylline in 500 ml of normal saline for a child (10 years old, 30 kg) suffering from acute bronchial asthma at the rate of 1 mg/kg/hr. Aminophylline is available as 2.5% W/V in 10 ml ampoule.

_____

_____

_____

_____

_____

_____

_____

_____

_____

_____

_____

_____

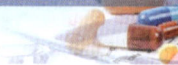

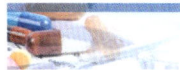

Date:

PRACTICAL 8

COMPETENCY

PH1.12: Calculate the dosage of drugs using appropriate formulae for an individual patient, including children, elderly and patient with renal dysfunction
PH2.4: Demonstrate the correct method of calculation of drug dosage in patients including those used in special situations

Objectives

At the end of this practical class, student should be able to:
- Calculate the dose for adults as well for paediatric patients
- Calculate the dose in case of renal disease
- Calculate loading and maintenance dose
- Calculate and understand drug dilutions and strength.

Domain: Skill
Level: Shows how
Teaching learning methods: Small group discussion, DOAP
Aligning assessment methods: Skill assessment, vivo voce
Number of procedure to be done independently for certification: None

Dose is the appropriate amount of a drug needed to produce a certain degree of response in a given patient. Recommended doses are based on the data of average adult patient. Doses of many drugs are not a simple linear function of body weight and age. Dose needs to be calculated in extreme side of age; means in both children and old age people and some special situations. Body surface area (BSA) is more appropriate and exact value method to which a children dose should be related. Body weight is most used for calculating the dose because it is easy method as compared to BSA.

Calculation of Doses

1. Adult and Children Dose

For a child weighing 55 kg and above, adult dose can be used. For other's doses need to be calculated. Dose of a drug is calculated as daily divided doses in mg/kg/day (solid), millilitre (liquid) or in IU (biological preparations).

Calculated dose = Adult dose × Weight (kg)/70   (On the basis of weight)
Calculated dose = Adult dose × BSA (m^2)/1.73   (On the basis of body surface area)

BSA is calculated using the following formula:

BSA (m^2) = HT (cm)$^{0.725}$ × BW (kg)$^{0.425}$ × 0.007184   (Dubois formula)
HT: Height, BW: Body weight, BSA: Body surface area

Child's dose as per age:

Child's dose = Adult dose × Age of child (years)/Age + 12   (Young formula)
Child's dose = Adult dose × Age in years/20   (Dilling's formula)

2. For Elderly Patients (>60 years)

There are no fixed rules or formulae for determining the dose in elderly patients. However, the dose may be reduced to 2/3rd of the adult dose due to decrease in renal/liver function and lean body weight. For example, aminoglycosides.

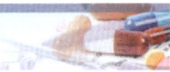

3. In Renal Failure

Few drugs are dependent on renal function for their elimination hence in patients with impaired renal function the dose of such drugs has to be reduced. For example, aminoglycosides, penicillins, cephalopsorins, etc. Calculation of dose for these patients is based on creatinine clearance and the following formula can be used:

$$\text{Calculated dose} = \frac{\text{Adult dose} \times \text{Creatinine clearance in renal insufficiency}}{\text{Creatinine clearance in normal individual}}$$

Creatinine clearance in a healthy individual of 70 kg (1.73 sq.m. BSA) = 100–120 ml/min.

Elimination includes excretion in urine, faeces, air, etc. and metabolism into different compounds (metabolites). It is expressed as volume per unit of time (ml/min.)

$$CL = CL \text{ renal} + CL \text{ hepatic} + CL \text{ other}$$

Clearance (Cl): Clearance of a drug is the theoretical volume of any body fluid from which the drug is completely removed in unit time.

4. Loading Dose

Few drugs with high apparent volume of distribution or long plasma half-life or in emergency have to be given in loading dose. Loading dose is the amount of drug given as initial dose or prime dose to achieve therapeutic plasma concentration.

Example: Chloroquine in malaria and lidocaine in arrhythmia.

Loading dose = Therapeutic plasma concentration x Vd (litre)

Apparent volume of distribution (Vd): It is the ratio between the total amount of drug in body (dose given) and the concentration of drug measured in blood or plasma.

$$Vd = \frac{\text{Total amount of drug in body (mg)}}{\text{Concentration in plasma (mg or mcg/litre)}}$$

Therapeutic plasma concentration: When rate of absorption is equal to rate of elimination. It takes approximately 4 to 5 half-life to reach this state.

Plasma half-life ($t_{1/2}$): It is the time taken for the plasma concentration to be reduced to half of its original value. It is determined by volume of distribution and clearance (elimination).

$$t_{1/2} = 0.693/\text{Kel} \quad \text{and} \quad Cl = \text{Kel} . Vd$$

5. Maintenance Dose

A maintenance dose may be required in some cases to maintain a steady state. After giving loading dose the amount of drug excreted is replenished daily and that is known as maintenance dose. This depends on the clearance of the drug.

Maintenance dose = Therapeutic plasma concentration × Clearance

Drug Dilutions and Strength

Strength of a drug is expressed in mg/g (solid), millilitre (liquid) or in IU (biological preparations), percentage or proportion.

Strength expressed as percentage

- For solids in liquid 1% solution means 1 gm of solute or active substance in 100 ml (10 mg/ml). (Weight in volume or W/V)
- For solids in solid means number of grams of active constituent in 100 gm of formulation (W/W)
- For liquid in liquid means the volume of the active constituent (in ml) in 100 ml of total formulation. (Volume by volume, v/v)

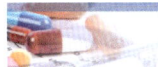

Strength expressed as proportion

1 : 1000 means 1 gm (1000 mg) of solute in 1000 ml of solvent (1 mg/ml)

Examples:

S. No	Ratio	Percentage (%)	Concentration
1.	1 : 100	1%	10 mg/ml
2.	1 : 1000	0.1%	1 mg/ml (1000 mcg/ml)
3.	1 : 10,000	0.01%	0.1 mg/ml (100 mcg/ml)
4.	1 : 1,00,000	0.001%	10 mcg/ml

Exercise: What amount of drug solution will you administer from a 5 ml of vial containing 10 mg of drug if the required dose is 2 mg?

Calculation

5 ml of the vial contains 10 mg,
i.e. 1 ml will contain = 2 mg
Hence 1 ml should be administered if 2 mg of the drug has to be administered

LET'S DO THIS

1. Calculate the dose for a 35 kg paediatric patient if adult dose for a 70 kg patient is 500 mg.

_____

_____

_____

_____

_____

2. What amount of drug solution will you administer from a 10 ml of vial containing solution of the strength of 2% of drug if the required dose is 20 mg?

_____

_____

_____

_____

3. What is the strength of 0.1% solution in mg/ml?

_____

_____

_____

_____

_____

4. If 1 ml of 1 : 2000 solutions is diluted up to 5 ml, what will be strength of resultant solution?

_____

_____

_____

_____

_____

5. Calculate the corrected dose in a patient with creatinine clearance of 50 ml/min, if drug is cleared 70% by kidney and 30% by liver and is normal therapeutic dose is 100 mg/day.

_____

_____

_____

_____

_____

6. What is the loading dose to achieve plasma concentration of 3 mg/L? Here, volume of distribution = 4.7 litres/hour, clearance = 20 litres

_____

_____

_____

_____

_____

7. The creatinine clearance of a patient with renal failure is 25 ml/min. How would you adjust the normal dosage of gentamicin for this patient. (dose of gentamicin 80 mg three times a day).

_____

_____

_____

_____

_____

_____

_____

_____

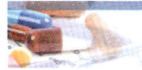

EXPERIMENTAL PHARMACOLOGY

Date:

Introduction to experimental pharmacology

Objectives

At the end of this practical class, student should be able to:
- Define experimental pharmacology
- Enlist commonly used experimental animals
- Explain principle of three 'R'
- Explain computer assisted learning (CAL).

Domain: Know
Level: Knows how
Aligning teaching learning methods: Small group discussion
Aligning assessment methods: Witten, viva voce
Number of procedure to be done independently for certification: None

Experimental Pharmacology

Study of drugs in animals is known as experimental pharmacology. It is known as preclinical phase of drug development.

A number of new drugs are introduced every year and many new aspects of older drugs are found out. The development of a new drug after drug discovery phase starts with experiments on animals, i.e. preclinical development. Any new compound before it is accepted or used on human beings has to meet strict safety and efficacy criteria which have to submit during regulatory approval. This drug discovery and development process is broadly divided into four parts:

1. Drug discovery phase (therapeutic concept—target selection and validation—lead finding and optimization)
2. Pre-clinical development (in animals)
3. Clinical development (clinical trials phase I/II/III/IV in human beings)
4. Regulatory approval.

Animal Experiments are Carried Out to:

- Establish the actions of potentially useful compound to predict adverse and toxic effects in humans.
- Establish the safety of the drugs through toxicological studies.
- Establish pharmacokinetic properties of the drug.
- Find out dose range and to determine maximum recommended starting dose (MRSD) in humans.
- Study the actions of established drugs.
- Study of drug interactions.

Animal Experiments are of Two Types

In vitro experiments

They are carried out on isolated organs, tissues or cells maintained under physiological conditions. Physiological salt solutions are used to maintain physiological conditions which differ from tissue to tissue and animal to

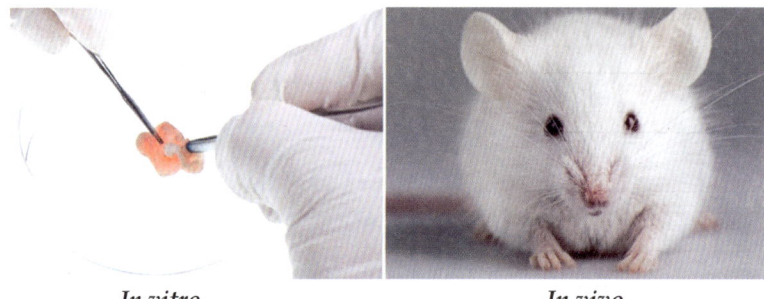

In vitro   *In vivo*

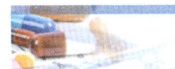

animal, and type of ions used in it. Physiological solution keeps the tissue alive for a longer period of time by providing nutrition, isotonicity and work as buffering agents. The action produced by drugs on isolated tissues is directly proportional to the drug dose and time of the exposure of tissue.

In vivo experiments

These are carried out on live, intact animals. These studies are useful in observing the response to a drug under the influence of several systems of the body.

Both *in vitro* and *in vivo* tests in animals are used to predict adverse and toxic effects in humans.

COMMONLY USED EXPERIMENTAL ANIMALS

Rodents (albino rats, mouse, guinea pigs, hamster), non rodents (rabbit, monkey, dog, cat, pig), miscellaneous (zebra fish, frog, pigeon) are the commonly used experimental animals because of firstly mammals (Rodents) are having close anatomical, biochemical and physiological similarities with humans. Secondly due to good reproduction capacity and short lifespan, the physiological and pharmacological actions of newer compounds/drugs will be easily examined at various stages/intervals. The Committee for the Purpose of Control and Supervision of Experiments on Animals (CPCSEA) is a statutory Committee, which is established under Chapter 4, Section 15(1) of the Prevention of Cruelty to Animals Act 1960. Permission from CPCSEA is required for conducting experiments involving use of large animals. Recently this committee is renamed as Committee for Control and Supervision of Experiments on Animals (CCSEA). In a book "The Principles of Humane Experimental Technique" published in 1959 by Russel WMS and Burch RL, the principles of so-called "Three R's" (Replacement, Reduction, and Refinement) were formulated.

Replacement—with alternative methods instead of proper experiments on animals

Reduction—of animals used keeping the validity of obtained results

Refinement—of animal experiment to minimize general suffering of the animal and suppress or eliminate pain.

COMPUTER ASSISTED LEARNING (CAL)

Since animal experiments involve pain, suffering, and in some cases sacrificing the animals, the use of animals in experimental pharmacology for demonstration/teaching purposes has now been restricted from increasing ethical issues. Various non-animal alternatives of teaching and learning pharmacology experiments have been designed and developed along with the advances in computer technology.

Computer assisted learning is a new concept in experimental pharmacology for undergraduates. Using computer simulations as an alternative to animal experiments allows a greater advantage of lesser involvement of time, effort, repeatability and prevents the unethical killing of animals. Computer assisted learning is almost similar to the experimental model of learning. The CAL software is designed in such a way to simulate animal experiments by demonstrating the effect of various drugs on animal tissues and the student can view and even perform them which give him/her a chance to have hands on experience with these virtual experiments. Both *in vitro* and *in vivo* correlations can be made with the help of the user friendly software's.

LET'S DO THIS

1. Write name of two lower animals in which animal experiments can be conducted without the permission of CPCSEA.

   _____

   _____

   _____

   _____

   _____

2. Write full form of CCSEA.

_____

_____

_____

3. Write rule of three "R".

_____

_____

_____

_____

_____

_____

_____

_____

_____

4. True/False
    i. *In vitro* experiments are conducted in live intact animals.
    ii. Phase I trial is conducted in animals.

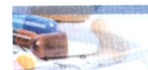

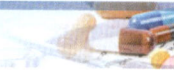

Date:

PRACTICAL 10

COMPETENCY PH4.1

Administer drugs through various routes in a simulated environment using mannequins

Objectives

At the end of this practical class, student should be able to:

- Describe precautions during administration of drug through various routes
- Explain withdrawal of drug from vial and ampoule
- Demonstrate the important steps in administration of injections by intradermal, subcutaneous, intramuscular and intravenous routes in mannequins
- Demonstrate method of administration of parenteral infusions.

Domain: Skill
Level: Shows how
Teaching learning methods: DOAP
Aligning assessment methods: Skill assessment, OSPE with checklist, viva voce
Number of procedure to be done independently for certification: None

Materials Needed

Syringe, drug to be administered, needle (as per the route), liquid disinfectant, cotton wool, adhesive tape, tourniquet and simulator.

There are various routes through which drugs are administered in our body. Many routes do not required assistance like oral, sublingual route, etc. but parenteral routes require various aseptic precautions and assistance. For administration of drugs; syringes and needles (as per route) are required in parenteral routes. These are also required to withdraw secretions from the body.

Syringes

Syringes are available in the capacity of 1 to 50 ml and have graduation marks on the barrel. Special insulin syringe have graduation marks in units. They are made up of plastic or glass. The glass syringe can be reused after sterilization. Plastic syringes are disposable and are commonly used with disposable needles. Prefilled syringes are meant for single administration. Example typhoid vaccine, anti-D immunoglobulin, etc.

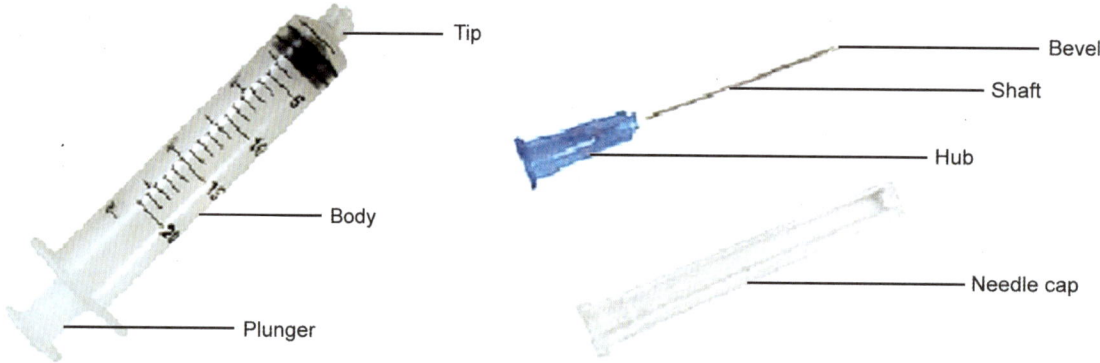

Needles

The needles are made up of metal and consist of hub which locks to the syringe tip. They are available in different sizes as per the length and the outer diameter of the shaft (gauge). Needles are almost always disposable. The diameter varies from 13 gauge (thickest) to 27 gauge (finest). The thick or large bore needles are used for thick or oily liquids. For example, benzathine penicillin.

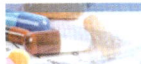

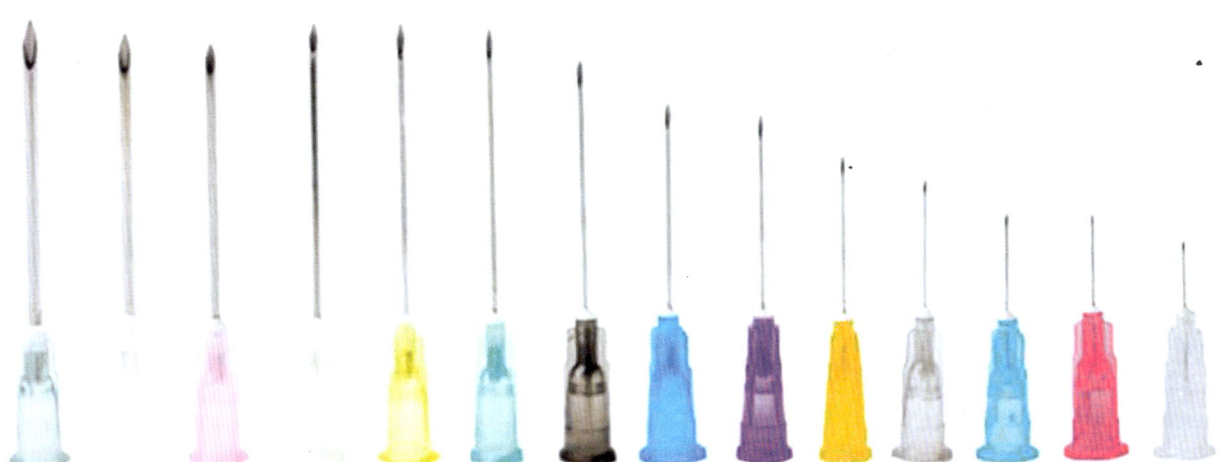

The commonly used parenteral routes with needles sizes are shown below:

Route	Gauge	Syringe	Site of injection
Intradermal	24–26	Tuberculin syringe	Anteromedial surface of forearm
Subcutaneous	24–25	Tuberculin or insulin syringe	Loose subcutaneous tissue of skin, outer surface of arm, front of thigh
Intramuscular	20–24	2–5 ml	Deep between muscle mass, deltoid, dorsogluteal, ventrogluteal (adults), lateral femoral (children)
Intravenous	18–22	Intra catheter	Anterior cubital vein, other veins at the elbow
Intracardiac	14–16	10 ml	Through 4th intercostal space into the chamber of the ventricle
Intra-articular	18–19	10 ml	Joint space

Precautions to be Taken while Administering an Injection

1. Observe aseptic precautions
2. Clean site of injection with germicidal solution.
3. Use sterile equipment.
4. Apply proper technique to minimize pain and chances of injury to the nerves and vessels.
5. Select the appropriate size of syringe and needle.
6. Syringe and needle should be empty before use.
7. Always check the label including expiry date of drug.
8. Disinfect the tip and rubber cap of vial.
9. Mix only compatible drugs.
10. Never return unused drug to stock bottle.
11. Avoid needle prick injury.
12. Destroy needle and syringe safely. Do not reuse disposable syringes and needles.
13. Do not touch anything with needle once its protective cover is removed.
14. Do not prick yourself or anyone other with the used needle.
15. Press sterile cotton onto the opening. Fix with adhesive tape.

Withdrawal of Drug from Ampoule

1. Put needle on syringe, without touching their tips.
2. Remove liquid from the neck of the ampoule by flicking it or swinging it fast in a downward spiraling movement.
3. Protect your fingers with gauze if ampoule is made of glass.
4. Break the neck of ampoule and split it off.
5. Aspirate drug from ampoule.
6. Remove air from the syringe.

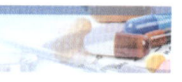

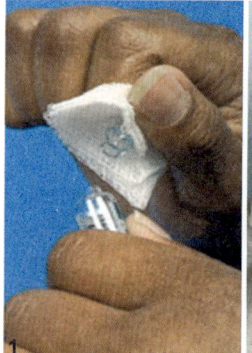 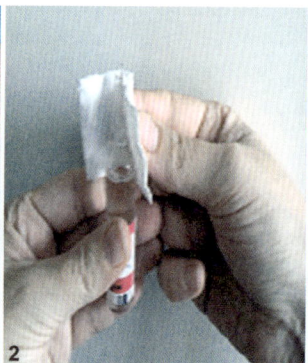 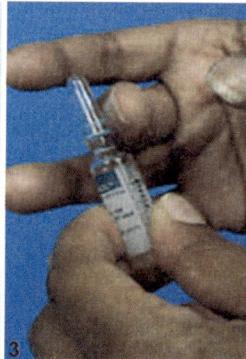 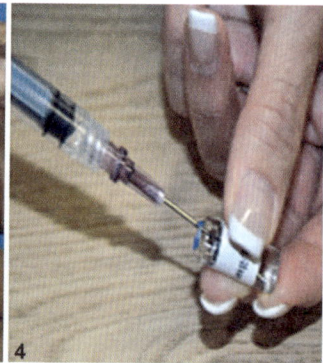 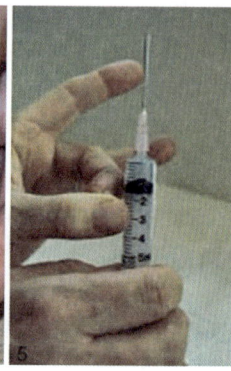

Withdrawal of Drug from Vial

1. Disinfect the rubber cap of vial.
2. Use syringe with volume twice the amount of solution required.
3. Place needle on syringe, without touching their tips.
4. Suck as much air into the syringe as the volume of solution to be injected.
5. Insert needle into the top of vial.
6. Turn it upside down.
7. Pump air into vial.
8. Withdraw appropriate amount of drug.

Dissolving a Drug in a Medium

1. Insert needle with syringe containing medium into vial.
2. Hold it in upright position.
3. Inject fluid into vial and turn it upside down.
4. Shake the vial well.

Technique for Intradermal Injection (id)

1. Observe aseptic precautions.
2. Reassure the patient and explain the procedure.
3. Uncover the area to be injected (inner surface of the forearm and the upper back) and disinfect skin with germicidal solution like spirit.
4. Pinch the skin. Insert needle intradermally at an angle of 5–15 degrees and release skin.
5. Inject slowly (0.5–2 minutes).
6. Bleb formation will occur.
7. Withdraw the needle swiftly.

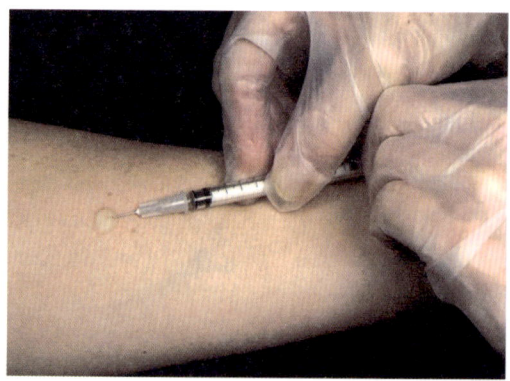

Technique for Subcutaneous Injection (SC)

1. Observe aseptic precautions.
2. Reassure the patient and explain the procedure.
3. Uncover the area to be injected (upper arm, upper leg, and abdomen) and disinfect skin.
4. Pinch and fold the skin. Insert needle in the base of the skin fold at an angle of 30–45 degrees and release skin.
5. Aspirate briefly; if blood appears, withdraw needle, replace it with new one, if possible and start again from disinfecting the skin.
6. Inject slowly (0.5–2 minutes)
7. Withdraw needle quickly.

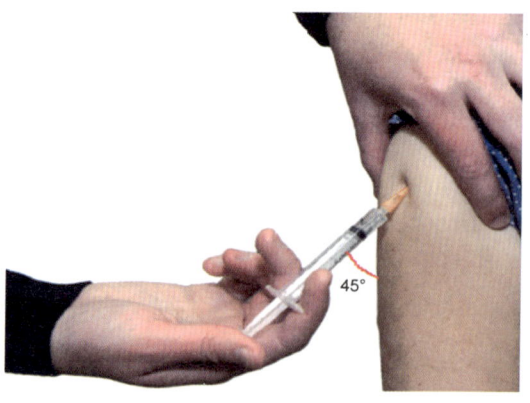

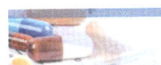

Technique for Intramuscular Injection

1. Observe aseptic precautions.
2. Reassure the patient and explain the procedure.
3. Uncover the area to be injected (lateral upper quadrant major gluteal muscle, lateral side of upper leg, deltoid muscle) and disinfect.
4. Ask patient to relax the muscle.
5. Insert needle at an angle of 90 degree. Watch depth.
6. Aspirate briefly; if blood appears, withdraw needle, replace it with new one, if possible and start again from disinfecting the skin.
7. Inject slowly (0.5–2 minutes).
8. Withdraw the needle swiftly.

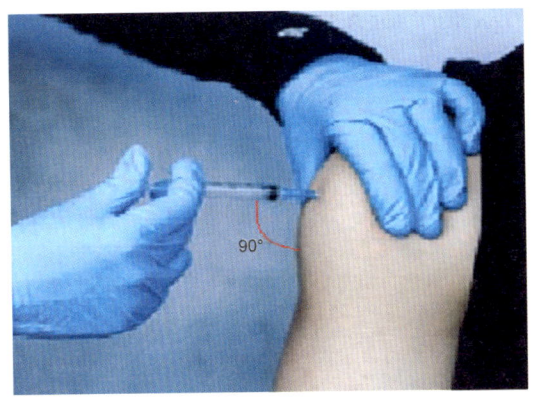

Technique for spinal injection

1. Observe aseptic precautions.
2. Reassure the patient and explain the procedure.
3. Patient is given a proper position—sitting or lateral.
4. Insert the spinal needle in L3–L4 or L4–L5 interspace.
5. Once the needle is in its appropriate space, remove stylet and cerebrospinal fluid can be seen at the needle hub.
6. Once confirmed, inject the local anaesthetic drug alone or with adjuvant slowly.
7. Needle is then removed carefully and discarded.
8. Patient should be laid in lateral tilt position and allowed to stabilize.
9. Continuous monitoring of vitals required.
10. Surgical procedure can be commenced once anaesthetic effects have kicked in.

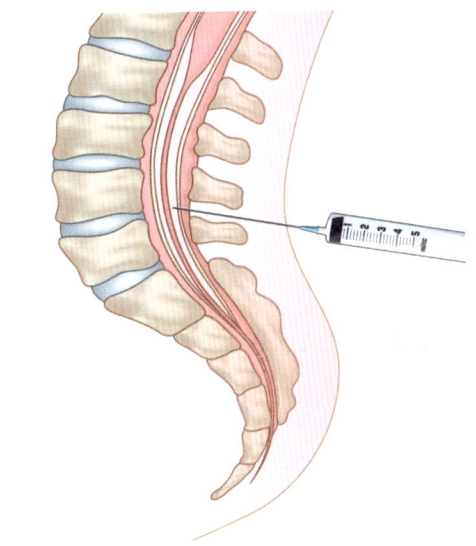

Technique for Intravenous Injection

1. Observe aseptic precautions.
2. Reassure the patient and explain the procedure.
3. Uncover the arm completely.
4. Ask the patient relax and support his arm below the vein to be used. Apply tourniquet and look for suitable vein. Wait for the vein to swell.
5. Stabilize the vein by pulling the skin taut in the longitudinal direction of the vein. Do this with the hand you are not using for inserting the needle.
6. Insert needle at an angle of 35 degrees.
7. Puncture skin and move needle slightly into the vein (3–5 mm).
8. Hold the syringe and needle steady.
9. Aspirate; if blood appears, hold the syringe steadily as you are in the vein. If it does not come, try again.
10. Loosen tourniquet.
11. Inject very slowly.

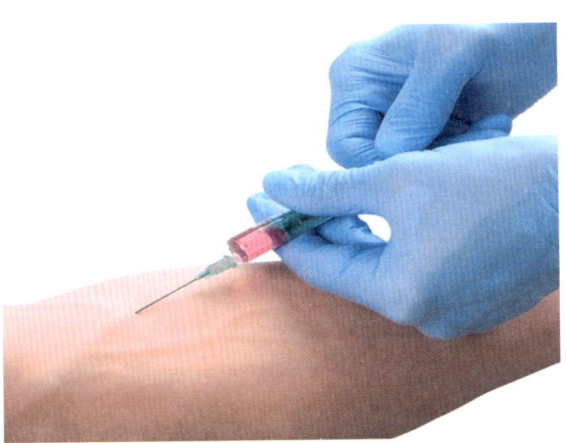

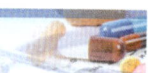

Equipment for Administering an Intravenous Infusion

a. IV cannula
b. IV infusion set—it consists of following parts:
   1. Insertion spike—it is used to be fixed in the IV fluid bottle.
   2. Plastic tubing—it is for passage of fluids.
   3. Drip chamber (Murphy's chamber) with filter (for blood transfusion) or without filter—It is used to fix the drop rate.
   4. Control clamp or roller—it is used to control rate of flow.
   5. Latex tube—it is used for injecting additional drugs.
   6. Needle adapter—it is to be introduced inside the needle.

Method of Administration of Intravenous Infusions

1. Select a proper vein and make it prominent by applying a tourniquet.
2. Pull the skin in longitudinal direction of vein.
3. Insert the cannula at an angle of 35 degree.
4. Puncture the skin, move the needle horizontally in vein.
5. Slowly remove the stylet of cannula.
6. Loosen the tourniquet.
7. Secure the cannula with adhesive tape.
8. Connect cannula to IV set through needle adapter.
9. Adjust the flow rate as required.

LET'S DO THIS

1. What is angle at which needle should be inserted in case of intramuscular injection and intradermal injection?
_____
_____
_____
_____
_____

2. Identify the picture. Write its one advantage.
_____
_____
_____
_____
_____

3. What are the steps for withdrawal the drug from ampoule?
_____
_____
_____
_____

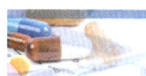

4. Identify route of drug administration in this picture and write two drugs given by this route.

_____

_____

_____

_____

_____

_____

_____

_____

5. Match the following.
   Needle Gauge_____Route
   26   IV
   24   IM
   18   ID
   20   Intra articular

6. Inject 1 ml of drug intramuscularly in a given simulator. (Assessment by checklist of steps)

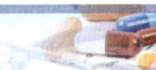

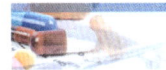

Date:

PRACTICAL 11

COMPETENCY PH4.2

Demonstrate the effects of drugs on blood pressure (vasopressor and vasodepressors with appropriate blockers) using computer aided learning.

Objectives

At the end of this practical class, student should be able to:
- Enlist various vasopressor, vasodepressors and their blockers with their mechanism of action on blood pressure
- Demonstrate the effect of various drugs on blood pressure (BP) in a simulated environment.

Domain: Skill
Level: Shows how
Teaching learning methods: Through computer assisted laboratory, DOAP
Aligning assessment methods: Skill assessment, viva voce
Number of procedure to be done independently for certification: None

Materials Needed

Computer assisted laboratory, computer with dog blood pressure software

In 2nd year pharmacology practical classes are conducted to demonstrate the effects of drugs on the blood pressure (BP) on dog's experiment. Experiment on large animals requires permission from the Committee for Control and Supervision of Experiments on Animals (CCSEA). This experiment has replaced by simulating it on a computer using Computer Assisted Learning (CAL) software. Animal experiment using CAL software is sufficient to meet the objectives of a practical class for undergraduate students in pharmacology.

Procedure

The software displays a simulated chart recorder on which the animated tracings of BP are recorded continuously. The student/teacher/demonstrator can choose any drug (and the dose) from the already given list in the software, administer it to the virtual dog and measure its effects on BP.

Drugs	Dose (μg/kg)	Drugs	Dose (μg/kg)
Adrenaline	2–5	Propranolol	1 mg
Noradrenaline	2–5	Acetylcholine	1–5
Isoprenaline	2–5	Atropine	0.5 mg
Ephedrine	1 mg	Histamine	0.2–5

There are two modes of experiment; tutorial and examination mode. When the software is run under the tutorial mode, it allows the student to test all the drugs in the given list and observe their effects and discuss them. In the examination mode, an unknown drug is given and the student is asked to find out its nature by comparing its effects with those of known drugs.

EFFECT OF VARIOUS DRUGS ON BLOOD PRESSURE

- Any change in the blood flow towards carotid bodies or stimulation of a nerve causes a reflex action which leads to change in neurotransmitter levels at effector organs. This results in changes in blood pressure (BP) and/or heart rate (HR) and respiration.
- **Adrenaline (A):** On sudden rapid IV injection, it produces biphasic response. There is a marked increase in both systolic as well as diastolic BP (at high concentration, α_1-receptor mediated response predominates which lead to vasoconstriction). After this, a small vagal notch is observed due to vagal stimulation. It returns to

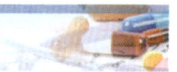

normal within a few minutes and a secondary fall in mean BP follows. The mechanism is rapid uptake and dissipation of adrenaline after that concentration around the receptor is reduced and this low concentration are not able to act on α_1-receptors but continue to act on β_2-receptors. The effect on respiration is variable initially with an increased respiratory rate followed by transient apnoea (due to reflex inhibition of respiratory centre).

- *Dale's vasomotor reversal:* Adrenaline administration after phentolamine (α-blocker) will act only on β_2-receptors to cause fall in BP and increase in heart rate through reflex action (No biphasic response).

- *Dale's vasomotor re-reversal:* Adrenaline administration after propranolol (β-blocker) will act only on α_1-receptors to cause a sharp rise in BP and increase in heart rate through reflex action (No biphasic response).

- **Noradrenaline (NA):** It causes rise in systolic, diastolic and mean BP. However, there is no vasodilatation (no β_2-action). So, peripheral resistance increases due to α-action. Its effects on respiration is insignificant.

- **Isoprenaline:** It decreases the BP due to predominant β_2-action. Their effect on respiration is similar to adrenaline.

- **Ephedrine:** It has direct as well as indirect actions on α and β receptors. Repeated administration of ephedrine produces a gradual and sustained decrease in BP. It fails to elicit the same pressure response on repeated administration. This phenomenon is known as tachyphylaxis or acute tolerance. Its effects on respiration are similar to adrenaline. It directly stimulates the respiratory centre.

Tachyphylaxis: Repeated administration of ephedrine produces a gradual fall in BP. It causes NA release from sympathetic nerve terminals and thus rises in BP. Frequent administration of ephedrine at short intervals leads to progressive depletion of NA stores in nerve terminals causing a progressive decrease in response to ephedrine.

- **Acetylcholine:** It stimulates M3 receptors on endothelium. Its stimulation causes quick vasodilatation by NO (diffuses quickly in the adjacent smooth muscles and rapidly cause vasodilatation) and the net effect is vasodilatation resulting in decreased BP. Acetylcholine is an agonist whereas atropine is an antagonist to muscarinic receptors.

Nicotinic action of acetylcholine: High dose of Ach given after atropine causes tachycardia and rise in BP due to stimulation of nicotinic receptors in sympathetic ganglia and release of catecholamines. Because vasculature does not possess parasympathetic supply, the effect of sympathetic stimulation will only be seen, i.e. rise in BP and heart rate.

- **Histamine:** Function and effect of H1 receptors on blood vessels is similar to M3 receptors. They are present on vascular smooth muscles and cause fall in BP due to slow vasodilatation by releasing endothelium dependent relaxing factor (EDRF). Persistent fall in BP is also due to H2 receptor (directly on vascular smooth muscle). Histamine is a non-selective agonist whereas mepyramine is H1 antagonist and cimetidine is H2 antagonist.

EXERCISES

Graph 1: Biphasic response of Adrenaline

Graph 2: Dale's Vasomotor Reversal

Graph 3: Dale's Vasomotor Re-reversal

Graph 4: Phenomenon of Tachyphylaxis

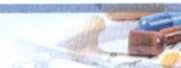

Graph 5: Nicotinic action of Acetylcholine

Graph 6: Effect of Histamine and Acetylcholine

LET'S DO THIS

1. Match the following:

Adrenaline	α_1, α_2 and $\beta_1, \beta_2, \beta_3$
Acetylcholine	α_1, α_2 and β_1, β_3
Noradrenaline	Muscarinic and Nicotinic
Isoprenaline	Indirectly acting drug
Ephedrine	$\beta_1, \beta_2, \beta_3$

2. Which receptors on sympathetic ganglia are responsible for releasing catecholamine? Explain.

_____

_____

_____

_____

_____

3. Following graph shows effect of drug A, B, and C on dog blood pressure. The responses of drug A, B, C are repeated after administration of propranolol (Shown as arrow in graph). Identify the probable nature of drug C giving reasons.
Drug A= Adrenaline (2.0 µg/kg)
Drug B= Noradrenaline (2.0 µg/kg)
Drug C= ??
Reason:

_____

_____

_____

_____

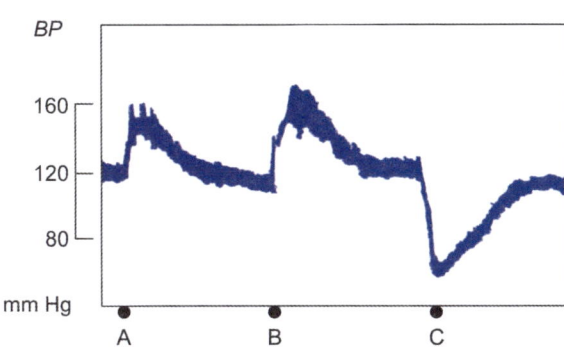 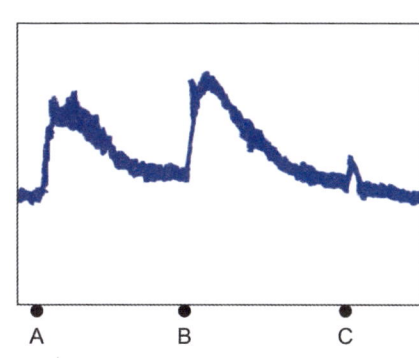

4. Following graph shows the effect of drug A and B on dog blood pressure. The response of drug A and B are repeated after administration of chlorpheniramine. Read the graph; identify the probable nature of drug B giving reasons.
Drug B = ??
Reason:

_____

_____

_____

_____

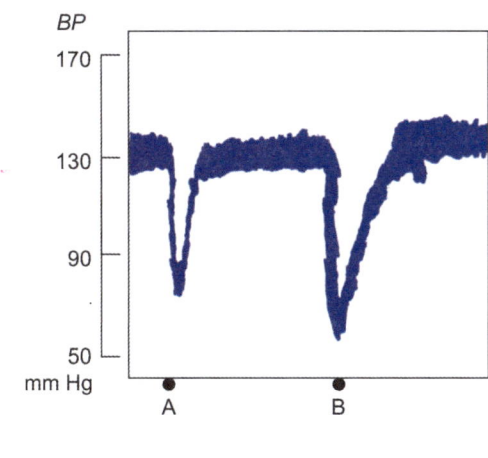 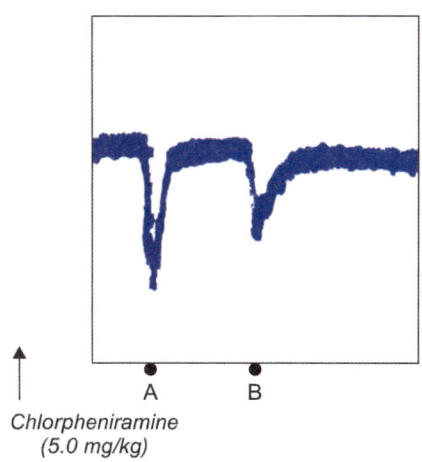

A: Acetylcholine

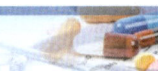

5. Following graph shows the effect of drug A, B and C on dog blood pressure. The responses of these drugs are recorded after administration of priscol (Tolazoline). Identify the probable nature of drug A and B giving reasons.

Drug A = ??

Drug B = ??

Drug C = Isoprenaline   (2.0 μg/kg)

Reason:

_____

_____

_____

_____

_____

_____

_____

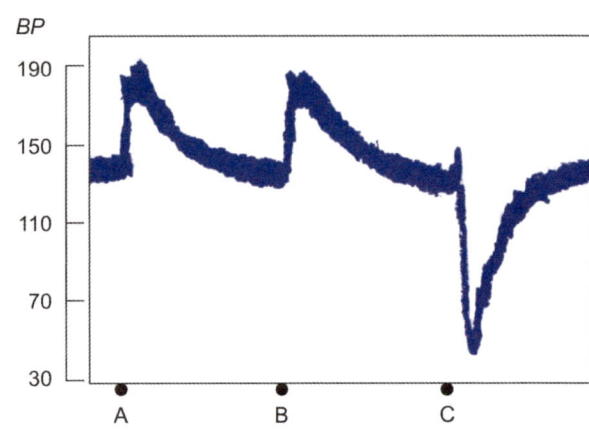

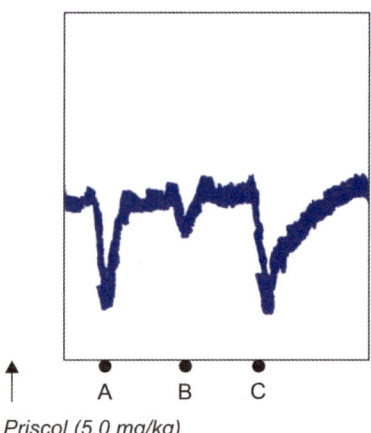

Priscol (5.0 mg/kg)

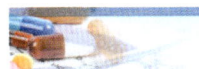

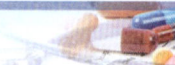

CLINICAL PHARMACOLOGY

COMPETENCY PH1.64

Describe overview of drug development, Phases of clinical trials and Good Clinical Practice.

Objectives

At the end of this practical class, student should be able to:
- Define clinical pharmacology
- Explain all the phases of clinical trial
- Explain other important aspects of clinical trial
- Explain principles of good clinical practice.

Domain: Knowledge
Level: Knows how
Teaching learning methods: Small group discussion
Aligning assessment methods: Written, viva voce
Number of procedure to be done independently for certification: None

Clinical Pharmacology

It is the scientific study of drugs in human being. It includes pharmacodynamic and pharmacokinetic investigation in healthy volunteers and in patients.

The drug discovery and development process is broadly divided into four parts:

1. Drug discovery phase (therapeutic concept → target selection and validation → lead finding and optimization)
2. Preclinical development (in animals)
3. Clinical development (clinical trials phase I/II/III/IV in human beings)
4. Regulatory approval.

After preclinical studies of experimental drug, studies in human beings are conducted as clinical trial. There are four phase of clinical trial. Each phase is considered a separate trial and, after completion of a phase, investigators are required to submit their data for approval from the FDA before continuing to the next phase.

Phase	Subjects	Aim	Dose	Number of participants
Preclinical	Animals	Testing of drugs in animals to gather efficacy, toxicity and pharmacokinetic information	Unrestricted	not applicable
Phase 0 (Micro dosing study)	Normal healthy volunteers	Pharmacokinetics	Very small, sub-therapeutic	10
Phase I (Human pharmacology)	Normal healthy volunteers (or patients of cancer, HIV, etc.)	Testing of drug on healthy volunteers for dose-ranging, pharmacokinetics, adverse events	Often sub-therapeutic, but with ascending doses	20–100
Phase II (Therapeutic exploration)	Patients	Testing of drug on patients to assess efficacy and safety	Therapeutic dose	100–500
Phase III (Therapeutic confirmation)	Patients	Testing of drug on patients to assess efficacy, effectiveness and safety	Therapeutic dose	500–3,000
Phase IV (Post marketing surveillance)	Patients with different age groups and gender	Adverse events or toxicity	Therapeutic dose	10000+

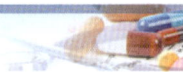

THE PRINCIPLES OF ICH-GCP

1. Clinical trials should be conducted in accordance with the ethical principles that have their origin in the declaration of Helsinki, and that are consistent with GCP and the applicable regulatory requirement(s).
2. Before a trial is initiated, foreseeable risks and inconveniences should be weighed against the anticipated benefit for the individual trial subject and society. A trial should be initiated and continued only if the anticipated benefits justify the risks.
3. The rights, safety, and well-being of the trial subjects are the most important considerations and should prevail over interests of science and society.
4. The available nonclinical and clinical information on an investigational product should be adequate to support the proposed clinical trial.
5. Clinical trials should be scientifically sound, and described in a clear, detailed protocol.
6. A trial should be conducted in compliance with the protocol that has received prior institutional review board (IRB)/independent ethics committee (IEC) approval/favourable opinion.
7. The medical care given to, and medical decisions made on behalf of, subjects should always be the responsibility of a qualified physician or, when appropriate, of a qualified dentist.
8. Each individual involved in conducting a trial should be qualified by education, training, and experience to perform his or her respective task(s).
9. Freely given informed consent should be obtained from every subject prior to clinical trial participation.
10. All clinical trial information should be recorded, handled, and stored in a way that allows its accurate reporting, interpretation and verification.
11. The confidentiality of records that could identify subjects should be protected, respecting the privacy and confidentiality rules in accordance with the applicable regulatory requirement(s).
12. Investigational products should be manufactured, handled, and stored in accordance with applicable good manufacturing practice (GMP). They should be used in accordance with the approved protocol.
13. Systems with procedures that assure the quality of every aspect of the trial should be implemented.

Most of the clinical trials are Double blind randomized control trial (RCT). Control may be placebo or standard drug. A placebo is an inactive pill, liquid, or powder which is pharmacological inert and has no treatment value. The placebo treatment should resemble the treatment under investigation in all respects. For example, shape, size, colour, frequency and duration of treatment. Blinding/masking is usually done to avoid bias. It can be single, double, triple.

Single blind: Study participant does not know the treatment he or she received

Double blind: Both study participant and investigator do not know the treatment group

Triple blind: Participant, investigator as well as statistician do not know the treatment group

Randomization

Randomization is usually done to avoid bias. Clinical trial may be randomized or nonrandomized, open or blind. Randomization minimizes the differences among group by equally distributing people with particular characteristics among all the trial subjects group. There are various randomization techniques and it is usually done by computer generated random numbers.

The Institutional/Independent Ethics Committee (IEC)

Group of scientific and non scientific members reviews the submitted researches plans (protocol), study design, confirms risk/benefit assessment, safety of the volunteers, etc. and approve/disapprove the initiation and conduct of the trial.

Informed Consent/Informed Consent Form (ICF)

Informed consent is a process whereby the patient/study participant voluntarily gives consent to participate in the study/trial after being adequately informed about the objective, nature, procedure, duration, associated risk and benefits, inconvenience that may be caused by participating in the study. ICF is a medicolegal document printed in the simple, understandable and non-technical language known to the participant, signed and dated personally by the subject and the investigator. If the participant is illiterate, an impartial witness (not related to the trial) should be present during the entire discussion and should sign the ICF. The volunteers should be given freedom for questions, discussion and allowed to refuse or withdraw from the study without penalty.

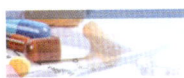

LET'S DO THIS

1. Can phase I study be conducted in Patients?

_____

_____

_____

_____

_____

_____

2. What do you mean by double blind clinical trial?

_____

_____

_____

_____

_____

_____

3. What is placebo?

_____

_____

_____

_____

_____

_____

4. Which phase of clinical trial is known as postmarketing surveillance?

_____

_____

_____

_____

_____

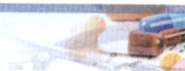

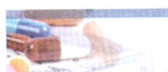

Date:

PRACTICAL 13

COMPETENCY

PH1.10: Describe parts of a correct, complete and legible generic prescription. Identify errors in prescription and correct appropriately.
PH3.1: Write a rational, correct and legible generic prescription for a given condition and communicate the same to the patient.

Objectives

At the end of this practical class, student should be able to:
- Define the term prescription
- Explain the meaning of rational prescription
- List all the parts of a prescription
- Explain importance of all the parts of prescription
- List the precautions while writing prescription
- Write the rational prescription for a given condition
- Appreciate the communication of prescription to the patient.

Domain: Skill and communication
Level: Performance
Teaching learning methods: Skill station with different diagnosis of the patients
Aligning assessment methods: Skill assessment, OSPE with checklist, viva voce
Number of procedure to be done independently for certification: 5

A prescription is a written order of a physician to a pharmacist to dispense medicines to a patient. It includes names and doses of the drugs, instructions for preparation and dispensing for the pharmacist and mode of administration for the patient. Literal meaning of prescription is "to write before" a drug can be prepared.

Rational Prescription

Rational prescription means use of the right drug for the right patient at the right time in the right dose and manner of administration, at affordable cost and with right information.

Steps for Rational prescription are
- Define diagnosis
- Specify therapeutic objectives
- Select appropriate drug/drugs/treatment on the basis of safety, efficacy, suitability and cost
- Start the treatment
- Give information, instructions as necessary
- Follow up of the treatment.

Prescriptions are of Two Types

Compounded

In this prescription the pharmacist prepares the medications according to the doses and dosage forms designed by the physician.

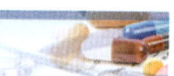

Example compounded prescription: Prescribe and dispense three doses of emulsion for an adult patient suffering from acute functional constipation.

Name of patient: Mr. XYZ

Age of patient: 33 Years

Sex: Male

Address: 23, Siddhi Apartments, Udaipur.

Name of Physician: Dr ABC

Qualification: MBBS

Address: 3, Prof. Quarters

Registration no: XXXX

Date: 03/03/2016

Diagnosis: Acute functional constipation

R_x

Castor Oil	8 ml
Gum Acacia	2 gm
Distilled Water ad	30 ml

Mft. Emulsio. Send such 30 ml.

Signa: Whole quantity to be taken in morning before breakfast.

Precaution: Shake well before use.

ABC

Regd. No. XXXX

Pre-compounded

Drugs prescribed are supplied by the pharmaceutical companies in ready prepared form by its non-proprietary or trade name.

Example pre-compounded prescription: Write a prescription for an adult patient suffering from enteric fever.

Dr ABC
MBBS
Address: 3, Prof. Quarters
Date: 03/03/2016
Diagnosis: Enteric fever

For, Mr. XYZ
Age: 33 Years, Gender: Male
Address: 23, Siddhi Apartments, Udaipur.

R_x

Tablet CIPROFLOXACIN 500 mg (14)
One tablet to be taken twice a day for seven days
Tablet PARACETAMOL 500 mg (5)
One tablet to be taken three times a day for first three days and then as and when required.

ABC
Regd. No. XXXX

Nowadays pre-compounded drugs (ready-made preparations marketed by pharmaceutical companies) are routinely prescribed. All prescriptions should be legible, unambiguous, dated and signed clearly for optimal communication between the prescriber, pharmacist, nurse and the patient. The prescriptions are generally written in English language.

Parts of Complete Prescription

1. Superscription
2. Inscription

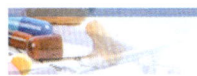

3. Subscription
4. Transcription/signatura/signa
5. Physician signature

Superscription

It consists of
- Name, qualification and address of the physician and the date
- Name, age, sex, address of the patient and the diagnosis

The physician's details are essential for the identity of the prescriber. Date helps in judging the interval between the issue of a prescription and that of dispensing it. The name and address of the patient are important to facilitate handling. From the age of the patient, the pharmacist can recheck the correctness of the dose prescribed.

The symbol 'R$_X$' stands for Latin recipe meaning "take thou of". The oblique line after R is considered as an ancient invocation of Chaldean physicians to Jupiter, the God of Health. It is a convention that all prescribers follow till date.

Inscription

It consists of
- Name of drug, its form (tablet, ointment, injection, etc.), strength, dose, routes, frequency of administration, duration and specific instruction to the patient.
- The International Nonproprietary (generic) name of the drug should be preferred over brand name. When more than one drug is prescribed, their order should be as follows:
  a. **Base:** It is a primary or principal drug for a particular clinical condition and should be written first. For example, an antimalarial drug.
  b. **Adjuvant:** It is a drug used to enhance/supplement the action of the basic drug and/or for any other associated symptom and it follows the base in serial order. For example, antipyretics in malaria.
  c. **Corrective:** It is a drug used to overcome any undesirable effect of the base or adjuvant. For example, antiemetic or antacid with antimalarial drug.
  d. **Vehicle:** Consist of an inert agent in which a drug is dispensed. It can be diluents, excipient or base.

Subscription

This is the direction to the pharmacist. For example, dispense 100 ml, send such number of tablets/capsules etc.

Transcription/Signatura: (Signa = Write or Label or Make)

This is the direction to the patients as how to take prescription. Renewal instructions and precautions should be written here. The prescriber indicate on every prescription order, whether it may be renewed and if so, how many times. It is very important for narcotics and other habit forming drugs to prevent its misuse.

Physician signature: It contains the signature of the physician with his or her registration number. Only the registered medical practitioner can prescribe the drug.

Common Prescribing Errors Include

- Poor handwriting
- Incorrect dose calculation for paediatric patients
- Prescriptions of drugs to which the patient is allergic (due to inadequate drug history)
- Overindulgence for multiple drug regimens, i.e. writing prescription orders for large quantities of medicines at a time especially controlled drugs unless such quantities are necessary
- Poor information furnished to patient
- Number of refills not specified
- No information about storage of drugs
- Undue high reliability on new drugs
- Writing Latin abbreviations which are difficult to decipher by the patient or pharmacist
- No cost consideration in selection of drugs, i.e. prescribing costly drugs unnecessarily

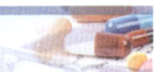

- Writing incomplete prescription in terms of drug dosage formulation, strength, dose, frequency, route, duration and instruction to the pharmacist and patient including date and signature
- Using abbreviated names of drugs and preparations
- Prescribing irrational drugs
- Giving insufficient, incomplete directions and instructions
- Signing blank prescriptions in advance
- Keeping prescription blanks in an open place
- Writing prescription orders for controlled drug in pencil or erasable ink
- Striking, scoring, overwriting and chemical formulae in the prescription.

Following care and Precaution Must be Taken while Writing Prescriptions

- Prescription orders are medicolegal documents. Therefore, they must be written legibly. The legal responsibility lies with the doctor who writes the prescription. Illegible prescription may create confusion or misinterpretation on the part of pharmacist/chemist/patient and result into medication errors and irrational use of medicines.
- Prescribing should be by generic name (in CAPITAL LETTER) as it will offer flexibility to the pharmacist in selecting the particular drug product and results into potential financial savings. Generics are usually cheaper than brand preparations.
- Full name of medicines should be used. Abbreviations such as PCM (paracetamol), etc. should not be used.
- It should be written in presence of patient without any hesitation. There should be no erasing, crossing out or tearing up of prescription in front of the patient.
- Prescription pad should be kept in safe custody.
- Never pre-signed the blank prescription.
- It is a legal document so it should be written by ink only.
- There should be no choice for the patient.
- Strength of the medication must be written in metric units.
  - Quantities of 1 gm or more should be written 1 gm, etc.
  - If less than 1 gm, it must be written in milligrams. For example, 500 mg not .5 gm
  - Avoid unnecessary zeros after decimal point. For example, 1 mg not 1.0 mg
  - There should be a space between number and its units. 10 mg not 10mg
  - When decimals are unavoidable, a zero must be written in front of the decimal point. For example, 0.5 ml not .5 ml
  - Use of decimal point is acceptable to express a range. For example, 0.5–1 gm
- The prescription must give clear, explicit and adequate instruction to the pharmacist and the patient on how to take the prescribed medicine. The phrases such as 'take as directed' should be avoided.
- Any non-pharmacological instructions like dietary advice and education on lifestyle changes should also be included in the prescription. Further, make sure that the patient has understood the instructions to improve the compliance and treatment outcome.
- There should not be a blank space between body of prescription and signature of doctor. If left blank strike off.

  A critical approach towards prescribing drugs not only avoids mistakes while dispensing drugs but also promotes rational use of drugs.

LET'S DO THIS

1. What is R_X?

_____

_____

_____

_____

_____

2. What are the contents of subscription?

_____

_____

_____

_____

_____

_____

3. What is the significance of age of the patient in prescription?

_____

_____

_____

_____

_____

_____

_____

_____

4. What is the significance of signature of the Doctor?

_____

_____

_____

_____

_____

_____

_____

5. What is Signa?

_____

_____

_____

_____

_____

_____

_____

_____

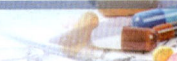

6. Write a rational, correct and legible generic prescription for 42-year-old male patient of acute attack of asthma and communicate the same to the patient

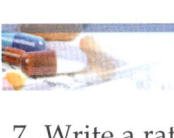

7. Write a rational, correct and legible generic prescription for a 46-year-old patient of type II diabetes mellitus and communicate the same to the patient

8. Write a rational, correct and legible generic prescription for an adult patient suffering from generalized tonic clonic seizures and communicate the same to the patient

9. Write a rational, correct and legible generic prescription for an adult patient suffering from upper respiratory tract infection and communicate the same to the patient

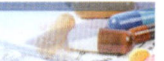

10. Write a rational, correct and legible generic prescription for an adult 36-year-old patient of Plasmodium Vivax malaria and communicate the same to the patient

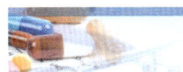

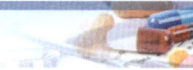

Date:

COMPETENCY PH3.2

Perform and interpret a critical appraisal (audit) of a given prescription.

Objectives

At the end of this practical class, student should be able to:
- Understand the steps of critical appraisal (audit) of prescription
- Evaluate the given prescription and rewrite the correct prescription.

Domain: Skill
Level: Performance
Teaching learning methods: Skill station with different prescriptions
Aligning assessment methods: Skill assessment, OSPE with checklist, viva voce
Number of procedure to be done independently for certification: 3

Word audit means official examination and verification of accounts or dealings as per dictionary but the audit in medical field focuses on 'evaluation of healthcare' and not on finances. Drug therapy is the core of medical practice but irrationality is common in this practice. More than 50% of medicines are prescribed, dispensed or sold inappropriately. 50% patients fail to take medicines correctly (WHO). Mushrooming of pharmaceutical companies and poor control by regulatory authority are also responsible for this practice in various means. To some extent this practice can be avoided by doing 'Prescription audit' which provide feedback to prescribers and other stakeholders.

Points to Remember while Doing Critical Appraisal (Audit)

- Format of the prescription—is it correct?
- Check out all the parts of prescription. Is any part missing?
- Is any abbreviations used?
- Is the aim of the treatment understood and fulfilled?
- Whether the diagnosis is recorded? Final or provisional.
- Is the drug prescribed appropriate as per the diagnosis?
- Is there over prescribing (Polypharmacy) or under prescribing?
- Whether drugs prescribed are by generic or/and brand names?
- Identify any ingredient/drug which is contraindicated/irrational but included in the prescription. Give reasons.
- Is there any unnecessary/irrational/hazardous drugs?
- Is there any irrational combination in prescription?
- Selection of the drugs depends on the diagnosis, specific characteristics of the patient, clinical presentation, laboratory test and cost of therapy. (Rational Prescription)
- Are the dosage, strength of medication, the dose, frequency, duration and route of administration (Safety and convenience) of drugs mentioned correctly? (Rational Prescription)
- Is there any ingredient which can result into drug interaction?
- Are the instruction, advice to the patient and pharmacist complete/correct?
- Is there any role of non-pharmacological treatment in the given clinical condition?
- Lastly whether prescription rational or irrational?

Example: Criticize (Audit) and rewrite the corrected prescription for an adult patient suffering from acute attack of gout.

    Tab Allopurinol 50 mg 1 tds
    Tab APC 500 mg 1 tds
    Patient is advised to take 1 glass of tomato juice along with drugs.

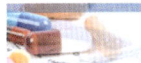

Criticism

- Form of prescription is not correct.
- Superscription, subscription, inscription and signature are missing.
- Abbreviations like APC should not be used.
- Allopurinol is not used in acute attack as it prevents formation of uric acid and it is not effective in controlling pain. It is more suitable for chronic gout.
- Duration of treatment is not mentioned.
- Tomato juice is avoided as it contains high uric acid concentration.

Corrected Prescription

Dr ABC

MBBS

Address Date:

Diagnosis: acute attack of gout

For Mr. XYZ

Age: Sex:

Address:

R$_X$

Capsule INDOMETHACIN 25 mg   (84)

2 tablets to be taken 2 times a day after meals for one week followed by one tablet to be taken 2 times a day for 4 weeks.

ABC

Reg. No. XXX

LET'S DO THIS

1. Criticize (Audit) and rewrite the corrected prescription for an adult patient of mild hypertension with Type II diabetes mellitus.
   Tab Metformin 100 mg BD
   Tab Amlodipine 5 mg OD for 7 days
   Tab Benzthiazide 25 mg ½ BD

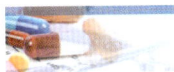
2. Criticize (audit) and rewrite the corrected prescription for an adult patient suffering from duodenal ulcer.
   Tab. Aspirin 100 mg 1 TDS
   Tab. Antacid 1 TDS
   Tab. Domperidone 50 mg

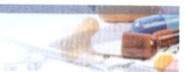

3. Criticize (audit) and rewrite the corrected prescription for an adult patient suffering drug induced Parkinsonism.
   Cap. Levodopa 10 mg daily
   Tab. Pyridoxine 5 mg

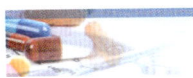

4. Criticize (audit) and rewrite the corrected prescription for young female patient suffering dysmenorrhea.
   Tab. Dicyclomine 100 mg
   Tab. Omeprazole 10 mg tds

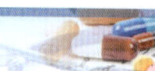

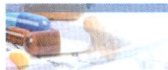

Date:

PRACTICAL 15

COMPETENCY PH3.3

Perform a critical evaluation of the drug promotional literature.

Objectives

At the end of the practical class the student should be able to:
- Define drug promotion
- Describe the different methods of drug promotion
- Enlist the essential contents of drug advertisements
- Critically evaluate a given drug advertisement.

Domain: Skill
Level: Performance
Teaching learning methods: Skill station with different sample of drug promotion literatures
Aligning assessment methods: Skill assessment, OSCE with checklist, viva voce
Number of procedure to be done independently for certification: 3

Materials Needed

Sample of various drug promotion literatures (drug advertisements).

All informational and persuasive activities by manufacturers and distributors, the effect of which is to influence the prescription, supply, purchase or use of medicinal drugs. (WHO)

The primary goal of the pharmaceutical industry is to promote a particular drug/product. So, the commercial source of information often emphasizes only the positive aspect of the product and gives little coverage to the side effects or adverse aspects. On the other hand, the drug promotional activities should provide scientific, correct, unbiased and critical information to the health professionals because physicians themselves report that they often use promotion as a source of information about new drugs and they have also not trained to deal with sales representatives.

Methods of Drug Promotion by Pharmaceutical Industries

1. Through drug advertisements in the professional journals, in the non-professional magazines or newspapers (for non-prescription drugs only), in drug information sheet to the clinician when a new product is introduced and via direct mail to physician.
2. Free drug samples to physicians
3. Promotion in scientific and educational activities, like seminars, conferences, etc.
4. Frequent visit by medical representatives to physician.

Drug Advertisements are of Two Types

- For new drug
- For old drugs (as reminder).

Contents of Drug Advertisements for New Drug

- Generic name(s) of the active ingredient(s).
- Brand name.
- Approved therapeutic uses.
- Dosage form or regimen.
- Side effects, major adverse reactions, precautions, contraindications, warnings.
- Major interactions.
- Name and address of manufacturer.
- References to scientific literature.

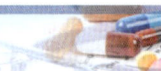

Content of Reminder Advertisement

After 4 years of drug introduction an advertisement is considered to be a reminder, and such advertisements may contain abbreviated information as follows:

- Brand name.
- International non-proprietary (generic) name (INN).
- Name of active ingredients.
- Name and address of manufacturer or distributor for the purpose of receiving further information.

WHO Criteria for Evaluation of Drug Promotion

1. Check the category of advertisement, whether it is for a new product or a reminder.
2. Check whether, brand name, generic or INN name of each ingredient, name and address of manufacturer, distributor is given or not.
3. Check for the following:
   - Amount of active ingredient(s) per dosage form or regimens.
   - Name of other ingredients known to cause problem.
   - Approved therapeutic uses.
   - Dosage form or regimen.
   - Side effects and major drug reactions.
   - Precautions, contraindications and warnings.
   - Major interactions.
4. *Check the claim:* If the advertisement contains some distinctive claims like 'the best', 'better', 'superior', etc. and always look for the basis of such claims.
5. Look for the catchy and exaggerated terms like 'antibiotic with excellent vision', 'speed with certainty', etc. which are usually meant to impress the prescriber.
6. Check the pictures and graphics used whether they are relevant to the product.
7. *Combination product:* If an advertisement promotes a combination product evaluate if there is any therapeutic advantage over the single substance.
8. Check the presentation of data: Whether data is presented in the form of bar, pie diagram, histograms, etc.
9. *Check the statistics:* Clinicians have limited knowledge and interest in statistics, so pharmaceutical company always takes the advantage of this ignorance.
10. Check the sample size, methods and statistical evaluation of the clinical trials quoted in the literature for their appropriateness and accurate interpretation.
11. *Check the references:* References published in old obscure or non indexed journals must be scrutinized. 'Symposium proceedings', 'data on file', 'in press', 'unpublished data', or 'personal communication', etc. should be evaluated with caution. Data of post marketing surveillance (PMS): If it is given, check whether it is misused for drug promotion. For example, 'free from side effects', 'no adverse effects found in PMS'.
12. Check whether all the required information is given or not under appropriate headings.

LET'S DO THIS

1. **Write two methods by which pharmaceutical companies advertise their product.**

   _____

   _____

   _____

2. **Critically evaluate a given drug advertisement on the basis of WHO criteria.**
   a. Type of promotional literature: (NEW/REMINDER)

   _____

   _____

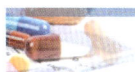

b. INN of drug (Yes/No):

_____

c. Brand name (Yes/No):

_____

d. Manufactures Address (Yes/No):

_____

e. Evaluate any missing information about drugs:
  • Amount of active ingredient(s) as per dosage form or regimens (Yes/No):

  _____

  • Name of other ingredients known to cause problem (Yes/No):

  _____

  • Approved therapeutic uses (Yes/No):

  _____

  _____

  _____

  _____

  • Dosage form or regimen (Yes/No):

  _____

  _____

  _____

  _____

  • Side effects (Yes/No):

  _____

  _____

  _____

  • Precautions, contraindications and warnings (Yes/No):

  _____

  _____

  _____

  • Major drug interactions (Yes/No):

  _____

  _____

  _____

f. Promotional claims (Yes/No):

_____

_____

_____

g. Catchy words (Yes/No):

_____

_____

_____

h. References are from standard medical journals (Yes/No):

_____

_____

_____

i. Visuals, graphs and illustrations used appropriately (Yes/No):

_____

_____

_____

j. Any other comments:

_____

_____

_____

k. Conclusion:

_____

_____

_____

3. **Critically evaluate a given drug advertisement on the basis of WHO criteria.**
   a. Type of promotional literature: (NEW/REMINDER)

   _____

   _____

   b. INN of drug (Yes/No):_____

   c. Brand name (Yes/No): _____

   d. Manufactures address (Yes/No): _____

   e. Evaluate any missing information about drugs:
      • Amount of active ingredient(s) as per dosage form or regimens (Yes/No):

      _____

      _____

      • Name of other ingredients known to cause problem (Yes/No):

      _____

      _____

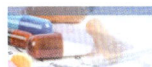

- Approved therapeutic uses (Yes/No):

  _____

  _____

  _____

- Dosage form or regimen (Yes/No):

  _____

  _____

  _____

- Side effects (Yes/No):

  _____

  _____

  _____

- Precautions, contraindications and warnings (Yes/No):

  _____

  _____

  _____

- Major drug interactions (Yes/No):

  _____

  _____

  _____

f. Promotional claims (Yes/No):

_____

_____

_____

g. Catchy words (Yes/No):

_____

_____

_____

h. References are from standard medical journals (Yes/No):

_____

_____

_____

i. Visuals, graphs and illustrations used appropriately (Yes/No):

_____

_____

_____

j. Any other comments:

_____

_____

_____

k. Conclusion

_____

_____

_____

4. **Critically evaluate a given drug advertisement on the basis of WHO criteria.**
   a. Type of promotional literature: (NEW/REMINDER)

   _____

   _____

   b. INN of drug (Yes/No): _____

   c. Brand name (Yes/No): _____

   d. Manufactures address (Yes/No): _____ _____

   e. Evaluate any missing information about drugs:
   • Amount of active ingredient(s) as per dosage form or regimens (Yes/No):

   _____

   _____

   • Name of other ingredients known to cause problem (Yes/No):

   _____

   _____

   • Approved therapeutic uses (Yes/No):

   _____

   _____

   _____

   • Dosage form or regimen (Yes/No):

   _____

   _____

   _____

   • Side effects (Yes/No):

   _____

   _____

   _____

   _____

- Precautions, contraindications and warnings (Yes/No):

  _____

  _____

- Major drug interactions (Yes/No):

  _____

  _____

f. Promotional claims (Yes/No):

  _____

  _____

g. Catchy words (Yes/No):

  _____

  _____

h. References are from standard medical journals (Yes/No):

  _____

  _____

i. Visuals, graphs and illustrations used appropriately (Yes/No):

  _____

  _____

j. Any other comments:

  _____

  _____

k. Conclusion:

  _____

  _____

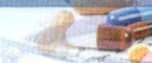

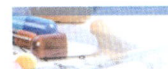

Date:

PRACTICAL 16

COMPETENCY

PH1.6: Describe principles of Pharmacovigilance and ADR reporting systems.
PH1.7: Define, identify and describe the management of adverse drug reactions (ADR).
PH3.4: To recognise and report an adverse drug reaction.

Objectives

At the end of the practical class, the student should be able to:
- Define ADR and other related terms
- Understand the importance of ADR monitoring
- Explain Pharmacovigilance Programme of India
- Learn the method of ADR reporting (i.e. how to report, when to report and whom to report an ADR
- Report an adverse drug reaction from a given case details in ADR reporting form.

Domain: Skill
Level: Shows how
Teaching learning methods: Small group discussion
Aligning assessment methods: Skill assessment, viva voce
Number of procedure to be done independently for certification: None

Materials Needed

ADR reporting Form, Patient's case records

Adverse drug reaction (ADR) is defined as "a response to a drug which is noxious and unintended, and which occurs at doses normally used in man for the prophylaxis, diagnosis, or therapy of disease or for the modification of physiological function."

Adverse drug event (ADE) is defined as "any untoward medical occurrence that may present during treatment with a medicine but which does not necessarily have a causal relationship with this treatment".

Medical error is "an unintended act (either of omission or commission) or one that does not achieve its intended outcomes." They are mishaps that occur during prescribing, transcribing, dispensing, administering, adherence, or monitoring a drug. For example, medication errors include misreading or miswriting a prescription.

Pharmacovigilance is the "science and activities dealing with the detection, assessment, understanding and prevention of adverse effects of drugs".

Types of ADRs

A. Augmented type—directly related to pharmacological action of drug. For example, hypokalaemia with digoxin
B. Bizzare type—idiosyncratic + genetically determined. For example, acute intermittent porphyria due to Sulphonamides in patients with G6PD deficiency.
C. Chronic type—associated with long-term use of drugs. For example, tardive dyskinesia with neuroleptics
D. Delayed type—teratogenicity or carcinogenicity
E. End of use—Abrupt stoppage of drug with corticosteroids
F. Failure of therapy—antibiotic resistance

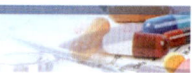

Why is there a Need to Report Adverse Drug Reactions?

1. The information collected during the pre-marketing phase of a drug is incomplete with respect to possible ADRs. Tests in animals do not always predict human safety. In clinical trials, patients are limited in number, the conditions of use differ from those in clinical practice and the duration of trials is limited. A good number of ADRs are evident when the drug is used on a large scale in uncontrolled situations for longer duration.

2. Information about rare but serious adverse reactions, chronic toxicity, and use in special groups (such as children, the elderly or pregnant women) or drug interactions is incomplete or not available and this can be obtained only through sustained vigilance.

Pharmacovigilance Programme of India (PvPI)

The Central Drugs Standard Control Organization (CDSCO), Directorate General of Health Services under the aegis of Ministry of Health and Family Welfare, Government of India in collaboration with Indian Pharmacopeia Commission, Ghaziabad has initiated a nation-wide Pharmacovigilance programme in 2004 for protecting the health of the patients by assuring drug safety. The programme is coordinated by the Indian Pharmacopeia Commission, Ghaziabad as a National Coordinating Centre (NCC). The PvPI National Coordinating Centre will collaborate with the WHO Collaborating Centre—Uppsala Monitoring Centre (UMC-Sweden) which runs for international drug monitoring with the coordination of national centres of various countries.

Objectives of PvPI

- To monitor Adverse Drug Reactions (ADRs) in Indian population
- To create awareness among healthcare professionals about the importance of ADR reporting in India
- To monitor benefit-risk profile of medicines
- Generate independent, evidence based recommendations on the safety of medicines
- Support the CDSCO for formulating safety related regulatory decisions for medicines
- Communicate findings with all key stakeholders
- Create a national centre of excellence at par with global drug safety monitoring standards.

ADR monitoring centres (AMC) are MCI approved medical colleges and hospitals, private hospitals and autonomous bodies like ICMR are included. The data obtained are entered in Vigi-Flow software. Vigi-Flow is a complete Individual Case Study Report (ICSR) management system created and maintained by the UMC. It is web-based and can be used as the national database for countries in the WHO Programme as it incorporates tools for report analysis, and facilitates sending reports to Vigi-Base. (The name of the WHO Global ICSR Database)

Spontaneous reporting is the reporting of ADRs by healthcare professionals to any suspected adverse drug reaction to a pharmacovigilance center and/or to the manufacturer. It is one of the important methods of collecting information about ADRs.

Who Should Report ADRs?

- All healthcare professionals. For example, general practitioners, specialists and all prescribers, pharmacists and other health workers
- Pharmaceutical manufacturers should report ADRs of their products to the competent regulatory authority
- Patients, patient's relatives or patients carers can also report.

What to Report?

All suspected adverse reactions, known or unknown, serious or otherwise should be reported. It is important to report even minor reactions of new drugs. For old established drugs, the reporting of serious ADRs is important. An increased frequency of a known ADR to a drug is also important.

Serious Adverse Drug Reactions

- Results in death
- Is life-threatening
- Requires inpatient hospitalization or prolongation of existing hospitalization
- Results in persistent or significant disability/incapacity or
- Is a congenital anomaly/birth defect

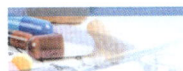
Whom to Report?

Adverse drug reactions may be reported to the respective nearest ADR Monitoring centre under the National Pharmacovigilance Programme, or directly to the CDSCO, New Delhi.

How to Report?

- Reporting is the process of providing ADR information by filling in the ADR form appropriately giving details of the clinical case as well as the ADR.
- Duly filled Suspected Adverse Drug Reaction Reporting Form can be send to the nearest Adverse Drug Reaction Monitoring Centre (AMC) or directly to the National Coordination Centre (NCC).
- Call on Helpline (Toll Free) 1800 180 3024 to report ADRs.
- Or can directly mail this filled form to pvpi@ipcindia.net or pvpi.ipcindia@gmail.com
- A list of nationwide AMCs is available at: http://www.ipc.gov.in, http://www.ipc.gov.in/PvPI/pv_home.html Notification

It is the process of informing any participating pharmacovigilance centre about the occurrence of a suspected ADR. The process may involve informing over telephone, in person, email, fax or any other means of communication-verbal or written. All notifiers must give their contact details so that the details of the ADR can be collected by the centre.

The ADR Reporting form

The ADR reporting form is used to notify a case report relating to a medical event (or laboratory abnormality) suspected to be induced by a drug.

Example:

- White Form issued by CDSCO (Central Drugs Standard Control Organisation, Government of India, New Delhi)
- Medwatch (US FDA)
- Yellow form (United Kingdom)
- Blue form (Australia).

Disadvantage of this voluntary reporting system through ADR forms is low reporting of ADR because of less involvement of doctors/participants due to it's voluntary and unpaid, Lack of awareness, busy schedule, inability to diagnosis of ADR, thinks that it's a prescribing error and lastly they thinks that someone else will report. Other systems are also used in various countries.

A case report of a suspected ADR should contain the following information:

1. The patient's age, sex and brief medical history (when relevant).
2. Description of the adverse reaction which includes:
   - Description (nature, localization, severity, characteristics)
   - Results of investigations and tests done, if any.
   - Start date, course and outcome of the event.
3. Suspected drug(s): name (brand or ingredient name + manufacturer), dose, route, start/stop dates, indication for use.
4. Details of all other drugs used (including self-medication).
5. Risk factors. For example, impaired renal function, previous exposure to suspected drug, previous allergies, social drug use.
6. Name and address of reporter.

CAUSALITY ASSESSMENT IN ADR MONITORING

It is a process of inference of a causal drug of an ADR through continuous assessment of information obtained from the case report.

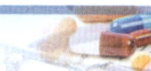

WHO-UMC Causality Categories

Definite/Certain	• Event or laboratory test abnormality, with plausible time relationship to drug intake • Cannot be explained by disease or other drugs • Response to withdrawal plausible (pharmacologically, pathologically) • Event definitive pharmacologically or phenomenologically (i.e. an objective and specific medical disorder or a recognized pharmacologic phenomenon) • Rechallenge satisfactory, if necessary
Probable/likely	• Event or laboratory test abnormality, with reasonable time relationship to drug intake • Unlikely to be attributed to disease or other drugs • Response to withdrawal clinically reasonable • Rechallenge not required
Possible	• Event or laboratory test abnormality, with reasonable time relationship to drug intake • Could also be explained by disease or other drugs • Information on drug withdrawal may be lacking or unclear
Unlikely	• Event or laboratory test abnormality, with a time to drug intake that makes a relationship improbable (but not impossible) • Disease or other drugs provide plausible explanation
Conditional/unclassified	• Event or laboratory test abnormality • More data for proper assessment needed, or • Additional data under examination
Unassessable/unclassifiable	• Report suggesting an adverse reaction • Cannot be judged because information is insufficient or contradictory • Data cannot be supplemented or verified

ADR reporting is the cornerstone pharmacovigilance activity. Physician should actively participate in this programme for patient safety. The following changes can occur after pharmacovigilance programme:

- Specific warnings about the product information
- Changing the legal status of a medicine. For example, from over-the-counter to prescription only
- In rare cases, removal of the medicine from the market, if the risks of a medicine are found to outweigh the benefits
- Rational use of medicines.

Prevention of ADRs by

- Following the steps of rational drug therapy
- Ruling out the history of previous drug reactions, allergic disease and possibility of drug interactions
- Correct drug administration techniques (vancomycin should give slow IV injection)
- Proper laboratory monitoring (PT in case of warfarin)
- Follow pharmacovigilance guidelines.

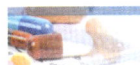

Exercise: Fill up the ADR reporting form based on the information provided in the patient's case record.

<table>
<tr><td>**Patient's Case Record**</td></tr>
</table>

Name of the patient: Mrs. Nita Patel

Age: 55 years

Sex: Female

Height: 5 feet, Weight: 70 Kg.

Hospital registration No: 646646

Date: 19/5/2017

Diagnosis: Upper respiratory tract infection

General physical examination: Patient healthy, well oriented in time and space, no jaundice, JVP normal

Vitals: HR—72/min

Respiratory rate—16/min

Temperature—38°C

BP 120/80 mm Hg

Systemic examination: Resp. system—normal   CVS—normal

Past history: No history of allergy, No recent of same complaint

Lab. investigation: Hb—12 gm% TLC—15000/cu mm

Treatment: given on 19/5/2017

Tab. Cotrimoxazole 480 mg twice daily for 6 days

Tab. Ibuprofen 400 mg thrice daily for 6 days

Advice: Salt water gargles for 5 days.

One day after treatment on 20/5/17, patient complaints of maculopapular rash and itching all over body. She was asked to stop Tab. Cotrimoxazole and prescribed Tab. Azithromycin 500 mg once daily for three days. She was also prescribed Tab. Cetirizine 10 mg once daily for 5 days and advised follow up after 1 week. After 1 week patient was better. Rashes disappeared. No other complaints.

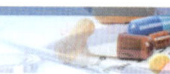

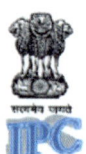

Version-1.2

SUSPECTED ADVERSE DRUG REACTION REPORTING FORM

For VOLUNTARY reporting of Adverse Drug Reactions by Healthcare Professionals

INDIAN PHARMACOPOEIA COMMISSION	FOR AMC/NCC USE ONLY
(National Coordination Centre-Pharmacovigilance Programme of India) Ministry of Health & Family Welfare, Government of India Sector-23, Raj Nagar, Ghaziabad-201002	AMC Report No. :
Report Type ☐ Initial ☐ Follow up	Worldwide Unique No. :

A. PATIENT INFORMATION	**12. Relevant tests/ laboratory data with dates**
1. Patient Initials _____ 2. Age at time of Event or Date of Birth _____ 3. M ☐ F ☐ Other ☐ 4. Weight_____Kgs	

B. SUSPECTED ADVERSE REACTION

5. Date of reaction started (dd/mm/yyyy)

6. Date of recovery (dd/mm/yyyy)

7. Describe reaction or problem

---

13. Relevant medical/ medication history (e.g. allergies, race, pregnancy, smoking, alcohol use, hepatic/renal dysfunction etc.)

14. Seriousness of the reaction: No ☐ if Yes ☐ (please tick anyone)

☐ Death (dd/mm/yyyy)   ☐ Congenital-anomaly

☐ Life threatening   ☐ Required intervention to Prevent permanent

☐ Hospitalization/Prolonged   impairment/damage

☐ Disability   ☐ Other (specify)

15. Outcomes

☐ Recovered   ☐ Recovering   ☐ Not recovered

☐ Fatal   ☐ Recovered with sequelae   ☐ Unknown

C. SUSPECTED MEDICATION(S)

S.No	8. Name (Brand/Generic)	Manufacturer (if known)	Batch No. / Lot No.	Exp. Date (if known)	Dose used	Route used	Frequency (OD, BD etc.)	Therapy dates Date started	Date stopped	Indication	Causality Assessment
i											
ii											
iii											
iv											

S.No as per C	9. Action Taken (please tick)						10. Reaction reappeared after reintroduction (please tick)			
	Drug withdrawn	Dose increased	Dose reduced	Dose not changed	Not applicable	Unkn own	Yes	No	Effect unknown	Dose (if reintroduced)
i										
ii										
iii										
iv										

11. Concomitant medical product including self-medication and herbal remedies with therapy dates (Exclude those used to treat reaction)

S.No	Name (Brand/Generic)	Dose used	Route used	Frequency (OD, BD, etc.)	Therapy dates Date started	Date stopped	Indication
i							
ii							
iii							

Additional Information:

D. REPORTER DETAILS

16. Name and Professional Address:_____
_____

Pin:_____ E-mail_____
Tel. No. (with STD code)_____
Occupation:_____ Signature:_____

17. Date of this report (dd/mm/yyyy):

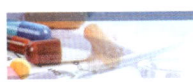

LET'S DO THIS

1. Expand the following abbreviations:
   i. PvPI_____

  ii. CDSCO–_____

  iii. AMC–_____

2. What is bizarre type of reactions? Write two drugs which lead to this type of reactions.
_____

_____

_____

_____

_____

_____

_____

_____

_____

_____

_____

_____

_____

_____

3. Identify the type of the ADR in this picture. Write one drug which shows this type of reactions.
_____

_____

_____

_____

_____

_____   Spinal cord

_____   Vertebra

_____   Dura meter

_____   Spinal fluid

_____

_____

_____

_____

_____

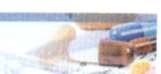

4. Identify the type of the ADR in this picture. Write one drug which shows this type of reactions.

_____
_____
_____
_____
_____
_____
_____
_____
_____
_____

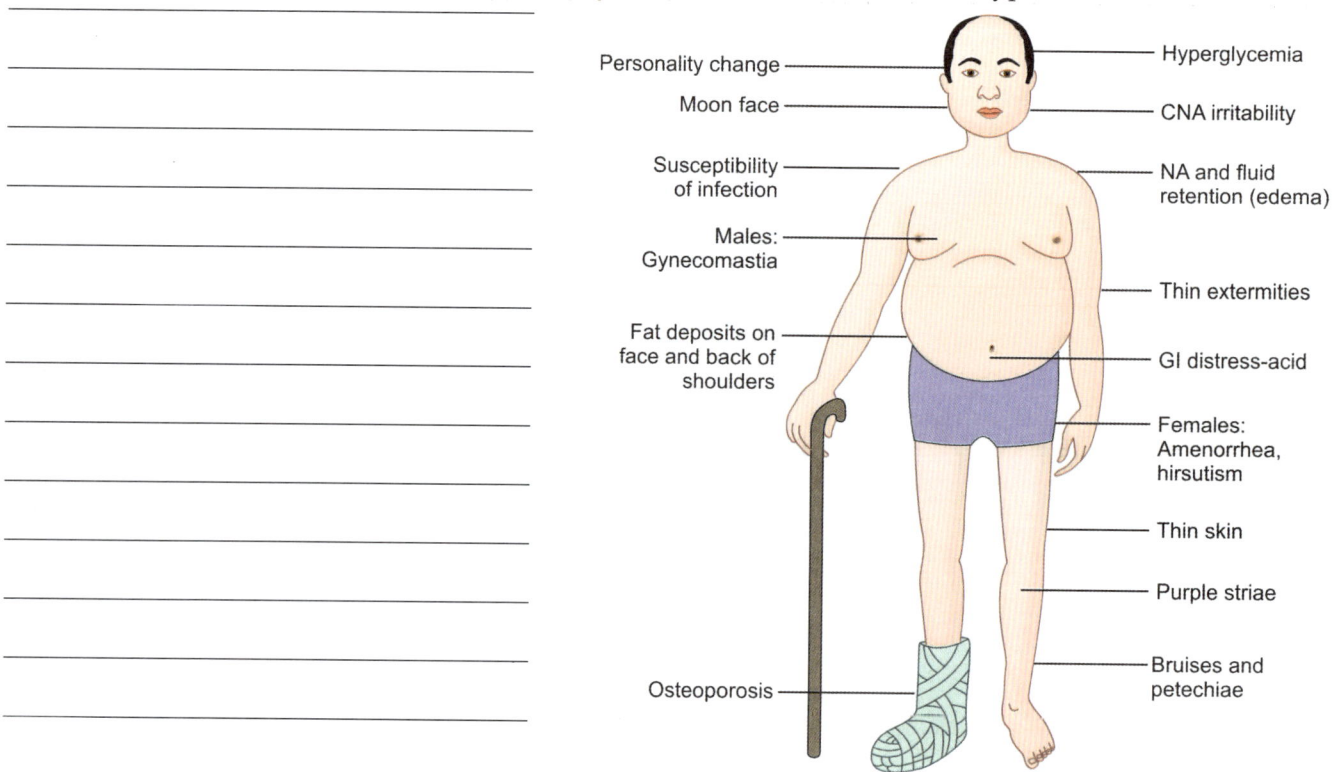

5. Fill the ADR form from the given case record of patient.

Patient's Case Record

Name of the patient: Kamal Kant Kumar

Age: 32 years

Sex: Male

Height: 6 feet,   Weight: 62 Kg.

Hospital registration No: xxxxx

Date: 2.10.18

Diagnosis: Essential hypertension

General physical examination: Patient healthy, well oriented in time and space, no jaundice, JVP normal

Vitals: HR—72/min

　　　　Respiratory rate—16/min

　　　　Temperature—Normal

　　　　BP 150/100 mm Hg

Systemic examination: Resp. system—normal   CVS—normal

Past history: No history of allergy, No family history of diabetes or hypertension

Lab. investigation: Hb—16 gm% TLC—6000/cu mm   Serum cholesterol—200 mg%

Treatment: given on 2.10.18

Tab. Prazosin   1 mg   Twice daily

Tab. Hydrochlorothiazide   25 mg Once daily

After 1 week treatment patient felt dizzy and fell down in the bathroom and sustained superficial scalp injury. The dose of Prazosin was reduced to 0.5 mg after checking the BP standing. (standing BP 100/70 mm Hg).

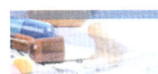

Version-1.2

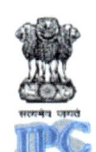

SUSPECTED ADVERSE DRUG REACTION REPORTING FORM

For VOLUNTARY reporting of Adverse Drug Reactions by Healthcare Professionals

INDIAN PHARMACOPOEIA COMMISSION (National Coordination Centre-Pharmacovigilance Programme of India) Ministry of Health & Family Welfare, Government of India Sector-23, Raj Nagar, Ghaziabad-201002	**FOR AMC/NCC USE ONLY**
	AMC Report No. :
Report Type ☐ Initial ☐ Follow up	Worldwide Unique No. :

A. PATIENT INFORMATION	**12. Relevant tests/ laboratory data with dates**

1. Patient Initials _____	2. Age at time of Event or Date of Birth _____	3. M ☐ F ☐ Other ☐
		4. Weight_____Kgs

B. SUSPECTED ADVERSE REACTION
5. Date of reaction started (dd/mm/yyyy)
6. Date of recovery   (dd/mm/yyyy)
7. Describe reaction or problem

13. Relevant medical/ medication history (e.g. allergies, race, pregnancy, smoking, alcohol use, hepatic/renal dysfunction etc.)

14. Seriousness of the reaction: No ☐ if Yes ☐ (please tick anyone)

☐ Death (dd/mm/yyyy)   ☐ Congenital-anomaly

☐ Life threatening   ☐ Required intervention to
                                                      Prevent permanent

☐ Hospitalization/Prolonged   impairment/damage

☐ Disability   ☐ Other (specify)

15. Outcomes

☐ Recovered   ☐ Recovering   ☐ Not recovered

☐ Fatal   ☐ Recovered with sequelae ☐ Unknown

C. SUSPECTED MEDICATION(S)										
S.No	8. Name (Brand/Generic)	Manufacturer (if known)	Batch No. / Lot No.	Exp. Date (if known)	Dose used	Route used	Frequency (OD, BD etc.)	Therapy dates		Indication	Causality Assessment
								Date started	Date stopped		
i											
ii											
iii											
Iv											

S.No as per C	9. Action Taken (please tick)						10. Reaction reappeared after reintroduction (please tick)			
	Drug withdrawn	Dose increased	Dose reduced	Dose not changed	Not applicable	Unkn own	Yes	No	Effect unknown	Dose (if reintroduced)
i										
ii										
iii										
iv										

11. Concomitant medical product including self-medication and herbal remedies with therapy dates (Exclude those used to treat reaction)

S.No	Name (Brand/Generic)	Dose used	Route used	Frequency (OD, BD, etc.)	Therapy dates		Indication
					Date started	Date stopped	
i							
ii							
iii							

Additional Information:	**D. REPORTER DETAILS**
	16. Name and Professional Address:_____ _____ Pin:_____E-mail_____ Tel. No. (with STD code)_____ Occupation:_____Signature:_____
	17. Date of this report (dd/mm/yyyy):

Confidentiality: The patient's identity is held in strict confidence and protected to the fullest extent. Programme staff is not expected to and will not disclose the reporter's identity in response to a request from the public. Submission of a report does not constitute an admission that medical personnel or manufacturer or the product caused or contributed to the reaction.

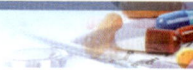

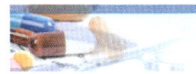
Date:

PRACTICAL 17

COMPETENCY PH3.5

To prepare and explain a list of P-drugs for a given case/condition.

Objectives

At the end of the practical class the student shall be able to:
- Explain/define concepts of P-drug and P-treatment
- Enumerate the steps for selection of P-drugs
- Prepare a P-drug for a given case.

Domain: Skill
Level: Performance
Teaching learning methods: Skill station with different cases/conditions
Aligning assessment methods: Skill assessment, OSPE with checklist, viva voce
Number of procedure to be done independently for certification: 3

Materials Needed

Standard pharmacology textbook and MIMS/IDR (or any other pharmaceutical indexing journal)

P-drugs are not what senior, colleague or teacher has suggested for particular disease, but these are those that have been chosen by the physician to be prescribed regularly for which they have become familiar along with the adverse effects of that drug and his/her priority choice for a given indication. It avoids repeated search for a good drug. The choice of P-drugs will differ from country to country and doctor to doctor because of varying availability and cost. P may mean Preferred, Personal, and Particular. It helps a prescriber to choose the most appropriate drug from a wide range available in the market. P-drug concept help in rational use of medicine in the form of right drug in right patient for right duration.

P-drugs are selected for a given patient with a certain clinical condition may not be always suitable for all the patients with the same condition. Hence, it is necessary to verify the suitability of P-drug for the patients with the high-risk factors like pregnancy, lactation, children, elderly, renal failure, hepatic failure, diabetes mellitus, etc.

P-treatment

All health problems may not always need drug treatment. They may be treated by simple advice, information and lifestyle changes. So P-treatment may not always include a P-drug. For example, dietary fibres for constipation.

Steps for Selection of P-drug are following

1. **Define the diagnosis:** Diagnosis of a disease from its signs and symptoms is necessary to select P-drugs.
2. **Specify the therapeutic objectives:** Therapeutic objectives should be clearly defined. For example, to decrease blood glucose, to reduce blood pressure, etc.
3. **Make a list of effective groups of drugs:** Two or more than two effective group of drugs for that diagnosis can be selected with the help of pharmacology textbook, reference book or hospital formulary.
4. **Choose an effective group according to criteria:** On the basis of efficacy, safety, suitability and cost of the treatment.

Efficacy	Safety	Suitability	Cost of treatment
This depends upon the both the pharmacokinetic and pharmacodynamic property of the drugs.	Side effects of different group of drugs are compared and a drug with fewer side effects is preferred.	Certain groups of patients like the elderly, children, pregnant women, those with kidney and liver diseases are high-risk groups and should always be considered carefully while selecting the P-drug. It should be selected with best convenient dosage form as per the diagnosis and dosage schedules for that particular disease.	Most cost effective drug should be chosen. The total cost of treatment is considered rather than cost per unit.

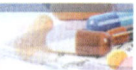

These criteria can be graded as −/±/+/++/+++ for efficacy, safety and suitability for all the groups by referring textbooks and cost can be check from IDR/CIMS/MIMS, etc.

5. **Choose a p-drug from effective group:** Same process just like groups; on the basis of efficacy, safety, suitability and cost of the treatment.

6. **Choose the p-drug, dosage form, dose schedule and duration of treatment:** The drug with suitable dosage form which is convenient to the patient should be selected. Recommended dosage schedules for all P-drugs can be found in formularies, physicians' desk references or textbooks of pharmacology and it should be based on patient condition. Duration of treatment depends upon type of disease like DM requires lifelong therapy and for treatment of bacterial infection 5 to 7 days therapy is required.

7. **Follow up the treatment:** Monitor the treatment through follow up is required for continue the same treatment or changes.

Exercise: Select a P-drug for a 62-year-old patient who was diagnosed to have angina pectoris and write a prescription.

Steps for Selection of P-drug

1. **Define the diagnosis:** Stable angina pectoris, caused by a partial occlusion of coronary artery
2. **Specify the therapeutic objective:** To reduce myocardial oxygen demand by decreasing preload, contractility, heart rate or afterload
3. **Make a list of effective groups:** These include
   a. Nitrates
   b. β-blockers
   c. Calcium channel blockers
4. **Choose a group according to criteria:**

Efficacy	Safety	Suitability	Cost*
Nitrates			
++	+	+++	Cheap
Beta-blockers			
++	+	+	Reasonable
Calcium channel blockers			
++	+	+	Reasonable

*Prototype drug cost amongst group can be compared for ease.

After comparing the three groups, nitrates are the group of first choice because, with acceptable efficacy and equal safety, they offer the advantages of an immediate effect by oral route and easy handling by the patient, at no extra cost. Injectable form of Beta blockers and CCB are required to produce immediate effect.

5. **Choose a P-drug from effective group (Nitrates):**

	Efficacy	Safety	Suitability	Cost
Glyceryl trinitrate	++	+	+	
Sublingual tab 0.5 mg				₹ 61.38/30 Tab.
Oral tab 2.6 mg				₹ 234/30 Tab
Isosorbide dinitrate	++	+	+	
Sublingual tab 5 mg				₹ 10.16/100 Tab
Oral tab 5 mg				₹ 42/50 Tab
Pentaeritritol tetranitrate	++	+	+	
Oral tab 10 mg				₹ 3.13/10 Tab
Isosorbide mononitrate	++	+	+	
Oral tab 10 mg				₹ 21.87/100 Tab

6. **Choose the p-drug, dosage form, dose schedule and duration of treatment**
   • *Choose p-drug and its dosage form:* In this case p-drug of choice for an attack of angina pectoris would be: sublingual tablets of glyceryl trinitrate 0.5 mg.

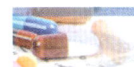

- *Choose a standard dosage schedule:* As the drug is to be taken during an acute attack, there is no strict dosage schedule. The drug should be removed from the mouth as soon as the pain is gone. If the pain persists, a second tablet can be taken after 5–10 minutes. If it continues even after a second tablet, the patient should be told to contact a doctor immediately.
- *Choose a standard duration of the treatment:* There is no way to predict how long the patient will suffer from the attacks, so the duration of the treatment should be determined by the need for follow-up.
7. **Follow up:** To monitor the treatment whether to continue the same treatment or changes in treatment are required.

Prescription

Dr ABC

MBBS

Address: 31, Kailash Apt.

Date: 28/04/2017

Diagnosis: Acute attack of angina

Mr. XYZ,

Age: 58 years Sex: Male

45, Ekinlignagar

Udaipur-313001.

R_X

    Tablet GLYCERYL TRINITRATE 0.5 mg   (3)

One tablet to be placed under the tongue. The tablet should be spitted off as soon as the pain subsides. If the pain does not subside it should be repeated after 5 minutes up to a maximum of 3 tablets.

ABC

Regd.No. XXX

LET'S DO THIS

1. What are the four criteria of choosing effective p-drug?

_____

_____

_____

_____

_____

_____

_____

_____

_____

_____

_____

_____

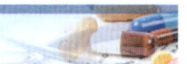

2. A 45-year-old male patient complains of occipital headache, heaviness and giddiness for 15 days. On repeated examinations, blood pressure was 150/96 mm Hg. Patient was diagnosed as having mild hypertension. Select a P-drug and write a prescription for the patient.

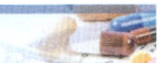

3. A 62-year-old male patient complains of loss of peripheral vision. After ophthalmic examination patient was diagnosed to have chronic open angle glaucoma. Select a P-drug and write a prescription for the patient.

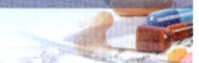

4. A young 24-year-old female complaining pain in both the loins radiating to the iliac fossae and suprapubic area, dysuria, turbid urine, fever 104°F with rigors. There is leucocytosis, urine acidic in reaction and shows presence of numerous pus cells, some red cells, epithelial cells and motile gram-negative bacilli. Select a P-drug and write a prescription for the patient.

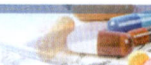

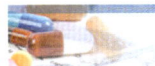

Date:

COMPETENCY PH3.6

Demonstrate how to optimize interaction with pharmaceutical representation to get authentic information of drugs

Objectives

At the end of the practical class the student should be able to:
- Enumerate different sources of drug information
- Demonstrate to get authentic information of drugs from pharmaceutical representation.

Domain: Skill
Level: Shows how
Teaching learning methods: Small group discussion, role play
Aligning assessment methods: Skill assessment, viva voce
Number of procedure to be done independently for certification: None

Materials Needed

Simulated medical representative.

Acquiring knowledge regarding drug is a dynamic process as new drugs due to arrival of new drugs and revealing of new indications and adverse effects in existing drugs after their utilization. So it is the duty of good professional to be aware about the changes and should know how to access authentic, up-to-date, unbiased and well documented scientific knowledge. There are many commercial and non-commercial sources of drug information which can provide large amount of drug related data within certain limits of their own. Hence a medical professional should be skilled for how to access and use judiciously the available information; depending on the type of information required.

Non-Commercial Sources

These provide educational and reliable information based on experimental evidence.
- Textbooks
- Drug compendia like Indian pharmacopeia (IP), British pharmacopeia (BP), etc.
- National formulary of India
- National list of essential drugs
- Good indexed journals with high impact factor
- Unsponsored CMEs, Seminar and Conferences
- Govt websites like www.cdsco.nic.in, www.fda.gov, etc.

Commercial Source

These are containing unverifiable statements and are persuasive to encourage drug use.

Information from pharmaceutical companies: These industries try to acquaint physicians about their products by contacting physicians by direct mailing and through medical representatives in form of brochures, by sponsoring and displaying their products in conferences, seminars and symposia and drug advertising in journals and websites.

Physician should ask for both positive and negative aspects of drug from medical representative (MR) with clinical evidences and references. He/she should then decide whether to prescribe that company drug or not. Pharmaceutical expenditures are rising rapidly, and entanglement between doctor and MR may influence doctors' behaviours which can lead to irrational prescription. To avoid this, doctors should not
- Accept direct gifts of equipment, indirect gifts through travel, or accommodation
- Accept samples of drugs for use by himself/his family members/relatives/friends. If accept them, he/she will use them only for needy patients

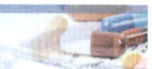

- Attend company sponsored courtesy-snacks/lunches/dinners and social or recreational events, continuing medical education, workshops, etc.
- Involve with or use of sponsored clinical guidelines.

LET'S DO THIS

1. Goodman and Gilman's Pharmacological Basis of therapeutics is which type of source of drug information.

2. Write two example of commercial source of drug information.

3. Write type of source of information for both sources.

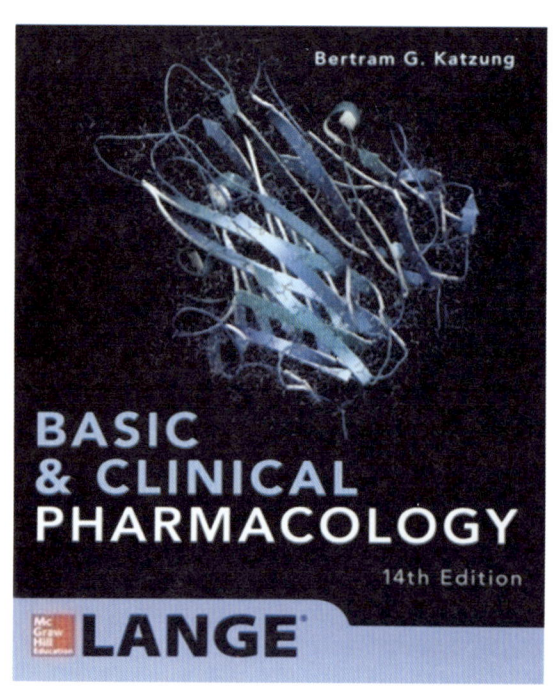

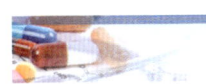

4. Comments on this scenario of Doctor interaction with MR.

   A medical representative came to visit for promotion of their pharmaceutical drug to Dr. Kailash from XXX Pharmaceutical company, with 50 sachet of their newly developed multivitamin, Y as free samples and claimed that this multivitamin will give good results in their patients. The company's representative also informed Dr. Kailash that if the medical store near his clinic received minimum 1000 prescriptions of this multivitamin every month, he would be given a free tour with his family anywhere in India. All the expenses would be borne by the pharmaceutical company. Dr. Kailash gave his patients this multivitamin only at ₹ 50/- per sachet, which was otherwise available in the market at a cost of ₹ 100/.

   _____

   _____

   _____

   _____

   _____

   _____

   _____

   _____

   _____

   _____

   _____

   _____

   _____

   _____

   _____

5. Perform role play in simulated environment with MR. Few students will observe and comments on the activity done. At the end teacher with give his/her suggestion to improve upon.

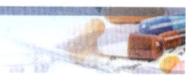

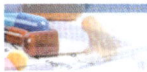

Date:

PRACTICAL 19

COMPETENCY PH3.7

Prepare a list of essential medicines for a healthcare facility

Objectives

At the end of the practical class the student should be able to:
- Define the essential medicines and appreciate its importance
- Describe the process of selecting essential medicines
- Prepare a list of essential medicine for a healthcare centre.

Domain: Skill
Level: Shows how
Teaching learning methods: Small group discussion
Aligning assessment methods: Skill assessment, viva voce
Number of procedure to be done independently for certification: None

Materials Needed

National list of essential medicines.

Essential medicines/drugs are those that satisfy the healthcare needs of the majority of the population. They should therefore, be available at all times in adequate amounts and in the appropriate dosage form. Essential drugs are an important component of promoting rational use of medicines.

The first 'Model list' of essential medicines was issued by WHO in 1977 and has been revised and updated from time to time. The WHO Model Lists of Essential Medicines has been updated every two years since 1977. The current versions are the 20th WHO Essential Medicines List (EML) and the 6th WHO Essential Medicines List for Children (EMLc) updated in March 2017.

Because of differences in the countries among incidence of disease and their pattern a uniform drug list is not feasible. For example, in New Zealand snakes are not found so antisnake venom which is an important essential medicine in Southeast Asian region, is not the part of essential list of New Zealand; therefore each country and state should prepare its own list as per their health needs, priority and disease pattern. However, the countries can use WHO list as a 'Model list'. Presently NLEM (National List of Essential Medicines of India) 2015 contains a total of 376 medicines of which 20 are FDCs. The selection of drugs should also be based on the level of healthcare centre, i.e. primary, secondary and tertiary.

EML must be reviewed from time to time (every 2–5 yrs) as there are changes in the disease pattern, emergence of drug resistance and development of better and safer drugs.

WHO Selection Criteria of an Essential Medicine

- The selection of drugs should be based on the experience rather than being opinion based.
- These medicines with long history of safety and efficacy determined by clinical studies should be included.
- Inclusion of newer drugs should be made only when these drugs offer any significant advantage over the existing ones.
- The quality, bioavailability and stability of the drugs should meet the set standards.
- Medicines with convenient dosage form and favourable pharmacokinetics that would ensure acceptability and compliance should be selected.
- In cases where two drugs bear close resemblance with respect to efficacy, stability, bioavailability, etc. Then
  - The drug which has thoroughly investigated should be selected.
  - The drug which has more appealing pharmacokinetic parameters should be selected.
  - The drug which can be prepared in appreciable quantity and quality at an affordable cost should be selected.

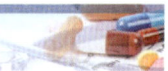

- **The cost: Benefit ratio** is an important criteria. Total cost of the treatment should be taken into consideration rather than unit cost of the drug.
- WHO maintains that the single drug or an active ingredient should find a mention in the EML. The fixed combination drugs should be mentioned only when they offer relatively better therapeutic efficacy, safety, patient compliance, etc. than the individual drugs.
- The periodic review of EML helps to incorporate significant new therapeutic advances and information if they offer distinct advantage over previously selected drugs. Drugs which are no longer found to be effective and safe can be replaced.

Advantages of Having EML

1. Promotes rational use of medicines.
2. The medicines will be easily accessible. It serves as a guide for procurement and supply of medicines in public sector.
3. Safe and effective medicines of good quality will be available.
4. Ensure that appropriate treatment will be available to the patients.

Orphan Drugs

Drugs that are used for the diagnosis, treatment or prevention of rare diseases are known as orphan drugs and disease is known as orphan disease. The overall cost incurred during development, manufacture and marketing of these drugs cannot be recovered by pharmaceutical company from selling the drugs but these drugs receive priority in drug approval process over other drugs during its trial. Government agencies also support the trials of orphan drugs. For example, acetyl cysteine, digoxin antibody, fomepizole, etc.

Emergency Medicines

These are life-saving medicines and require an immediate administration in a medical emergency. They can sustain life and/or prevent further complication and therefore should be available at all healthcare facilities, i.e. out patient departments, clinics, dispensaries and wards as well as primary (P), secondary (S) and tertiary (T) healthcare centres. Example paracetamol injection, diclofenac injection, atropine injection, adrenaline injection, isosorbide dinitrate sublingual tablets, ceftazidime injection, etc.

Example: Prepare an essential medicine list for an out patient department of a primary health centre in Udaipur district.

First step to find out the common problems encounter by an Indian Medical Graduate at this health centre: Suppose common problems are fever, malaria, vomiting, dehydration, abdominal colic, cut wound injury, cough, diarrhoea, bronchial asthma, malnutrition, anaemia, and amoebiasis.

Essential Medicines for PHC

Sr.No	Name	Formulation and strength
1.	Paracetamol	Tablet 100 mg, 500 mg
		Syrup 125 mg/5 ml
2.	Ibuprofen	Tablet 200 mg, 400 mg
		Injection 150 mg/ml
3.	Diazepam	Tablet 5 mg
		Injection 5 mg/ml in 2 ml ampoule
4.	IV fluids	5% Dextrose 500 ml, l liter
		Normal saline l liter
		Ringer lactate l liter
5.	Atropine	Injection 1 mg (as sulfate) in 1 ml ampoule
6.	Metoclopramide	Tablet 10 mg
		5 mg/ml in 2 ml ampoule
7.	Adrenaline Injection	1 mg (as hydrochloride) in 1 ml ampoule
8.	Salbutamol	Tablet 2 mg, 4 mg
		Aerosol 100 mcg per dose
		Injection 50 mcg/ml in 5 ml ampoule

Contd...

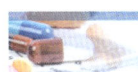

Sr.No	Name	Formulation and strength
9.	Glyceryltrinitrate	Tablet sublingual 500 mcg
10.	Surgical dressing	Povidone iodine ointment
11.	Lignocaine	Injection 1%, 2% vial
12.	ORS	Powder in sachet
13.	Ferrous sulphate	Tablet 200mg
14.	Metronidazole	Tablet 200 mg, 400 mg
		Oral liquid—200 mg/5 ml
		Injection—500 mg/100 ml
15.	Chloroquine	Tablet 150 mg
		Oral liquid—50 mg/ml

These selected essential medicines should be available at all times in adequate amounts and in the appropriate dosage form as per the number of patients daily coming to OPD.

LET'S DO THIS

1. Define essential drugs?

2. What are orphan drugs? Write two examples of it.

3. What is the rationale behind having a separate list of essential drugs in each healthcare facility?

4. Prepare an essential drugs list of cardiovascular drugs for a primary health centre.

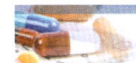

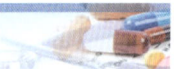

Date:

COMPETENCY

PH3.8: Communicate effectively with a patient on the proper use of prescribed medication
PH5.1: Communicate with the patient with empathy and ethics on all aspects of drug use
PH5.2: Communicate with the patient regarding optimal use of (a) drug therapy, (b) devices and (c) storage of medicines
PH5.3: Motivate patients with chronic diseases to adhere to the prescribed management by the healthcare provider
PH5.4: Explain to the patient the relationship between cost of treatment and patient compliance

Objectives

At the end of the practical class, the student should be able to:
• State the component of effective communication
• Realize and understand the importance of effective communication with the patient
• Communicate effectively regarding the proper use of a drug to improve patient compliance, drug adherence, storage of medicine in a simulated patient.

Domain: Attitude and communication
Level: Shows how
Teaching learning methods: Small group discussion, role play
Aligning assessment methods: Skill assessment, viva voce
Number of procedure to be done independently for certification: None

Materials Needed

Simulated patients, prescriptions.

Communication is the process for effective communication of sharing information or messages which ultimately leads to common understanding. It is derived from the Latin term 'communis' meaning common, but the information shared in a communication interaction is subject to difference in meaning. Communication is not so simple or straightforward and is hardly ever 100% successful. An effective communicator anticipates and plans for incomplete sharing of ideas. 7 'C' of effective communication are Complete, Clear, Courtesy, Consideration, Concise, Concrete and Correct.

Types of Communication

1. **Verbal:** This may be oral or written which illustrates various aspects of the clinical condition like diagnosis, prognosis and treatment including its cost. Though considered important part; constitutes only 7% of the communication.
2. **Para-verbal:** Includes tone, pitch, pacing, volume and accent of voice contributes to 38% of the communication.
3. **Non-verbal:** Non-verbal component forms 55% of the communication and includes expression in the forms of body language and other gestures like posture, appearance, facial expression, eye contact, body positioning and spatial distance which are not given due consideration but affects patients contentment and therapeutic results.

Three techniques (Conversational skills, Listening skills and Technical skills) are must to make communication effective. Doctor patient communication occurs while interviewing the patient during history taking, taking informed consent for a procedure, breaking the news (bad/good) and during management of the patient. Core communication skills are required during doctor patient communication are:

1. **Doctor–patient interpersonal skills**
   • Appropriate physical environment
   • Greeting patients

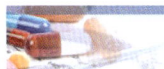

- Active listening and maintaining eye contact (during patients' complaints)
- Empathy, respect, interest, warmth and support
- Language
- Non-verbal communication
- Collaborative relationship
- Closing the interview.

2. **Information gathering skills**
   - Showing warmth in questioning style (questioning about complaints: length, severity)
   - Using an appropriate balance of open to closed question
   - Discuss personal and psychosocial issues of relevance
   - Silence, interruption and facilitation when needed
   - Clarify the information given by the patient (explanations to patient's questions)
   - Sequencing of events
   - Directing the flow of information
   - Summarizing.

3. **Information giving skills and patient education:**
   - Provide clear and simple information (diagnosis, explanation about diagnosis/disease)
   - Put important things first
   - Using repetition
   - Categorising information to reduce complexity
   - Using tools
   - Motivating patient adherence to treatment plans (explanation about treatment, particularly drugs)
   - Summarizing.

Communication during prescription to a patient is also necessary. Good communication about prescription to the patients can avoid irrationality to some extent. Irrationality can also due to patient's part because of following reason:

- Patients ask for quick cure (asking injection in place of oral treatment)
- Poor health education and wrong beliefs (taking too much dose for quick relief)
- Self-medication of other drugs without prescription
- Misinterpretation of information given on prescription
- Non-compliance (not taking complete course of therapy).

Physician should communicate to patient about prescription in detail for the following:

- Name of the drug
- Therapeutic effects as well as side effects
- How to take it
- Don't miss any dose as written in prescription
- If any problems occur while taking drug then he or she comes back to him/her
- Don't repeat the prescription without revisiting the doctor
- Don't stop treatment without consulting doctor and take medicine without missing single dose (patient compliance)
- Keep ready stock of your prescriptions in case of chronic diseases (drug adherence)
- Patient's questions about treatment
- How to prevent the disease/exacerbation
- Put medicines up and away and out of children's reach and sight at cool and dry place; make sure the safety cap is locked (storage of medicines)
- Cost of treatment
- Other relevant information.

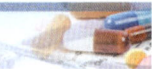

According to meeting of division of mental health, WHO held in Geneva 1993—Effective doctor–patient communication:

- Is an integral part of diagnosis.
- Enhance patient compliance to treatment plans.
- Contributes to doctor clinical competence and self assurance.
- Contribute to patient satisfaction.
- May contribute to cost and resource effectiveness.

Communication should not be cynical, misleading (giving false hope), creating guilt complex, accompanied with losing temper, and accompanied with negligence to patients emotions.

LET'S DO THIS

1. Write types of communication.

_____

_____

_____

_____

_____

_____

2. What do you mean by patients compliance?

_____

_____

_____

_____

_____

_____

3. Perform role play in simulated environment regarding the proper use of a drug to improve patient compliance in a simulated patient. Few students with observe and comments on the activity done. At the end teacher will give his/her suggestion to improve upon. (Various role play can be performed for different competency of communication).

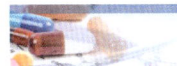

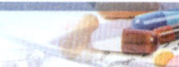

Date:

COMPETENCY PH1.8

Identify and describe the management of drug interactions

Objectives

At the end of this practical class, student should be able to:
- Describe different types of drug interactions
- Identify type of drug interaction in given conditions
- Manage the drug interactions.

Domain: Knowledge and skill
Level: Knows how
Teaching learning methods: Small group discussion
Aligning assessment methods: Written, viva voce
Number of procedure to be done independently for certification: None

Alteration in the effect of one drug due to the presence of another simultaneously administered drug is termed drug-drug interactions. Drug-drug interactions may be useful or harmful. Drug interactions are more common in presence of significant renal/hepatic impairment and in elderly patients because of multiple therapies for many chronic illnesses. Clinically significant drug-drug interactions may occur with when a drug is having narrow therapeutic index and due to microsomal enzyme induction and enzyme inhibition.

Types of Drug Interactions

1. *In vitro* **(outer side the body) drug interactions:** Interaction of one drug with another drug when they are mixed in the same syringe. They react chemically and can either lead to inactivation of that drug or precipitation
   Example:
   Thiopentone sodium + Succinylcholine
   Penicillin + Hydrocortisone
   Heparin + Hydrocortisone
2. *In vivo* **interactions (inside the body):** Can occur due to both pharmacokinetic as well as pharmacodynamic properties of the drug.

Pharmacokinetic Interactions

- **During absorption:** Due to chemical interaction of the drugs, altered gastric emptying or altered gut flora.
  Example: Antacids + Tetracycline
- **During distribution:** Due to displacement of drug from plasma protein binding site.
  Example: Warfarin + Sulfonamides
- **During biotransformation:** Due to microsomal enzyme induction or inhibition.
  Example: Phenytoin + Oral contraceptives
- **During excretion:** Due to altered urinary pH or interference with tubular secretion.
  Example: Penicillin + Probenecid

Pharmacodynamic Interactions

These interactions occur when two drugs act on the same or interrelated target resulting in additive/synergistic or antagonistic activities. For example, Alcohol+ Benzodiazepines.

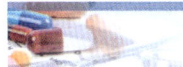

Examples: Common drug-drug interactions and their likely effect and reason (Various examples are taken from the book "Essentials of Medical Pharmacology" by Tripathi KD, 8th edition, 2021).

Precipitant drug	Object drug	Likely interaction and reason
Ampicillin and Amoxicillin	Oral contraceptives	Failure of contraception → due to interruption of enterohepatic circulation of the estrogen → reduction of gut flora; alternative contraceptive should be used
Ampicillin and Amoxicillin	Oral anti coagulants	Risk of bleeding → due to decreased vitamin K production in gut → Inhibition of gut flora; Monitor INR and reduce anticoagulant dose if needed.
Allopurinol	Ampicillin	Increased incidence of rashes → due to additive effect; Avoid concurrent use.
Allopurinol	6-Mercaptopurine Azathioprine	Risk of bone marrow suppression → due to inhibition of metabolism of object drug; Reduce dose of 6-MP/azathioprine.
Allopurinol	Warfarin Theophylline	Risk of bleeding → due to inhibition of metabolism of object drug; Monitor and reduce dose of object drug.
Aspirin and other NSAIDS	Sulfonylureas Phenytoin Valproate Methotrexate	Toxicity of object drug → due to displacement and/or reduced elimination; Avoid concurrent use or substitute NSAID with paracetamol.
Aspirin and other NSAIDS	Warfarin Heparin	Enhanced risk of bleeding → due to anti-platelet action and gastric mucosal damage; Avoid concurrent use.
Aspirin and other NSAIDS	ACEI'S Beta blockers Thiazides Furosemide	Reduced antihypertensive effect → due to inhibition of renal prostaglandin synthesis; Avoid concurrent use or substitute to other antihypertensive drugs
Carbenicillin Ticarcillin	Aspirin and other antiplatelet drugs	Risk of bleeding → due to perturbation of surface receptors on platelets → additive platelet inhibition; Avoid concurrent use.
Ceftriaxone Cefoperazone	Oral anticoagulants	Risk of bleeding → additive hypoprothrombinaemia; Monitor INR and reduce dose of anticoagulant.
Ciprofloxacin Norfloxacin Pefloxacin	Theophylline Warfarin	Toxicity of object drug → due to inhibition of metabolism; Monitor and reduce dose of object drug.
Clindamycin	Erythromycin Azithromycin Clarithromycin Chloramphenicol	Mutual antagonism of antibacterial action due to proximal binding sites on bacterial ribosomes.
Chloramphenicol	Warfarin Phenytoin Sulfonamides	Toxicity of the object drug → due to inhibition of metabolism; Avoid concurrent use
Cimetidine	Dicumoral	Enhanced bleeding tendency → due to inhibition of metabolism; Avoid concurrent use.
Carbidopa	L-DOPA	Increase the effect of L-DOPA due to inhibition of peripheral metabolism
Chronic alcoholism	Paracetamol	Hepatotoxicity → CYP2E1 enzyme induction lead to due to production of N-acetyl-p-benzoquinone; Avoid concurrent use
Diuretics	Tetracycline	Antianabolic effect of tetracycline increases urea production which is related to diuretics. Avoid concurrent use.
Diuretics	Lithium	Li+ toxicity → due to decreased excretion of Lithium; decrease the dose of Li+
Diuretics	Digoxin	Digoxin toxicity → Hypokalaemia caused by diuretic increases digoxin toxicity. Give K+ sparing diuretic/K+ Supplements.

Contd...

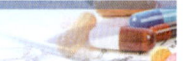

Precipitant drug	Object drug	Likely interaction and reason
Erythromycin Clarithromycin Ketoconazole Itraconazole Fluconazole Protease inhibitors	Terfenadine Astemazole Cisapride	Sevier ventricular arrhythmias → due to inhibition of metabolism by CYP3A4 → rise in blood levels of object drug; concurrent use is contraindicated.
Erythromycin Clarithromycin Ketoconazole Itraconazole Fluconazole Protease inhibitors	Phenytoin Carbamazepine Warfarin Sulfonylureas Diazepam Theophylline Cyclosporine HIV protease inhibitors	Toxicity of object drug → due to inhibition of metabolism by CYP3A4; Avoid concurrent use/readjust the dose of object drug.
Erythromycin Clarithromycin Ketoconazole Itraconazole Fluconazole Protease inhibitors	Statins	Higher risk of myopathy → Inhibition of Metabolism of statins; Avoid concurrent use.
Furosemide	Minocycline Aminoglycosides	Enhanced vestibular toxicity → additive ototoxicity and nephrotoxicity; Avoid concurrent use.
Gemfibrozil Nicotinic acid	Statins	Increased risk of myopathy → due to additive effect; Avoid concurrent use.
Iron salts Calcium salts Sucralfate Antacids	Tetracyclins Fluoroquinolones	Failure of antibiotic therapy → decreased absorption of antibiotics (object drugs) due to complex formation. Avoid concurrent use.
MAO- A inhibitors	Morphine	Severe respiratory depression due to inhibition of metabolism of morphine; Avoid concurrent use
Metronidazole Tinidazole Cefoperazone	Alcohol	Disulfiram-like reaction → Possibly due to accumulation of acetaldehyde. Warn the patient not to drink alcohol.
Metronidazole Tinidazole	Lithium salts	Lithium toxicity → due to decreased excretion; Monitor Lithium level and reduce lithium dose.
Metronidazole Tinidazole	Warfarin	Risk of bleeding → due to inhibition of metabolism; Avoid concurrent use.
NSAIDs	Ciprofloxacin and other Fluoroquinolones	Enhanced CNS toxicity, seizures; Avoid concurrent use.
Phenobarbitone Phenytoin Carbamazepine Rifampin	Metronidazole Doxycycline Chloramphenicol Protease inhibitors Warfarin Corticosteroids Sulfonylureas Oral contraceptives Antidepressants	Loss of efficacy of object drug → due to induction of metabolism; Avoid concurrent use or increase dose of object drug with monitoring.
Phenytoin	Vitamin D	Osteomalacia → due to enhanced metabolism of Vitamin D

Contd...

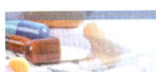

Precipitant drug	Object drug	Likely interaction and reason
Probenecid	Penicillin Ampicillin Cephalosporins	Inhibition of tubular secretion of object drugs → prolongation of antibiotic action; Desirable interaction utilized for single dose therapy.
Sulfonamides Cotrimoxazole	Phenytoin	Phenytoin toxicity → due to displacement and inhibition of metabolism; Avoid concurrent use.
Sulfonamides Cotrimoxazole	Warfarin	Risk of bleeding → due to displacement, inhibition of metabolism, and decreased production of vit K in gut; Monitor INR and reduce dose of warfarin.
Sulfonamides Cotrimoxazole	Sulfonylureas	Hypoglycaemia → due to displacement and inhibition of metabolism; Avoid concurrent use.
Sulfonamides Cotrimoxazole	Oral contraceptives	Failure of contraception → due to interruption of enterohepatic circulation of the estrogen → reduction of gut flora; alternative contraceptive should be used.
Tetracyclines	Oral contraceptives	Failure of contraception → due to interruption of enterohepatic circulation of the estrogen → reduction of gut flora; alternative contraceptive should be used
Tetracyclines Chloramphenicol Macrolides Clindamycin Cephalosporins	Penicillins	Bactericidal action of penicillins and cephalosporins may be antagonized by the bacteriostatic antibiotics.

LET'S DO THIS

1. A 40-year-old male patient was stable with warfarin therapy. He was prescribed fluconazole for fungal infection. What could be the possible interaction and why?

_____

_____

_____

_____

_____

_____

2. A 40-year-old male diabetic patient was stable on metformin for the last 1 year. He was prescribed chlorothiazide for Hypertension. What could be the possible interaction and how this can be avoided?

_____

_____

_____

_____

_____

3. A 60-year-old man takes sildenafil for erectile dysfunction. This patient was on nitrate treatment for coronary artery disease. What could be the possible interaction?

_____

_____

_____

_____

_____

_____

_____

4. Explain levodopa and pyridoxine interaction.

_____

_____

_____

_____

_____

_____

_____

5. Explain quinidine and digoxin interaction.

_____

_____

_____

_____

_____

_____

_____

6. Explain adrenaline and halothane interaction.

_____

_____

_____

_____

_____

_____

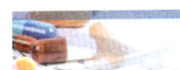

Date:

NOTES

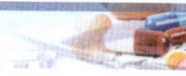

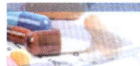

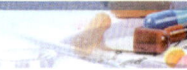

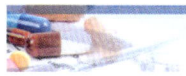

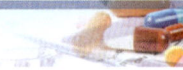

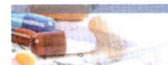

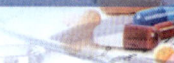

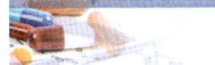

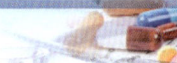

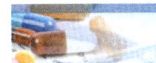

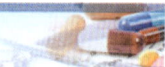

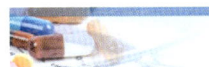

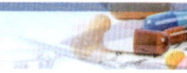

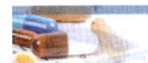

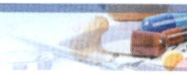

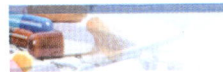

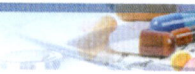

Annexures

EXAMPLES: FORMAT OF CHECKLIST FOR ASSESSMENT

To increase the objectivity of skill/communication assessment, preformed checklist can be used for all the practical or procedure in which various steps are required to perform activity.

Example 1: Checklist for Intradermal Injection

Sr. No.	Steps	Points
1.	Observe aseptic precautions	0.5
2.	Reassure the patient and explain the procedure	0.5
3.	Uncover the area to be injected (inner surface of the forearm and the upper back) and disinfect skin with germicidal solution like spirit.	1.0
4.	Pinch the skin. Insert needle intradermally at an angle of 5–15 degrees and release skin.	1.5
5.	Inject slowly (0.5–2 minutes)	0.5
6.	Bleb formation will occur	0.5
7.	Withdraw the needle swiftly	0.5
	Total	**5.0**

Example 2: Checklist for Use of Meter Dose Inhaler

Sr. No.	Steps	Points
1.	Take out the cap and clean the mouthpiece	0.5
2.	Shake the inhaler before use	0.5
3.	Exhale completely	1.0
4.	Place the mouthpiece between lips	0.5
5.	Tilt the head backward and press the inhaler while inhaling slowly and deeply	1.5
6.	Hold breath in inspiration for 10 seconds at least or as long as comfortable	0.5
7.	Gargles	0.5
	Total	**5.0**

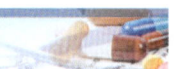

ABBREVIATIONS

Rational prescription should be written without using abbreviations but some abbreviations are still in use by doctors while prescribing drugs. These abbreviations if not correctly interpreted may lead to medication errors.

A. Time of Administration

Abbreviation	Latin (word)	English meaning
a.c.	ante cibum	before meals
p.c.	post cibum	after meals
i.c.	inter cibum	in between meals
o.d.	omni in die	once a day
b.i.d.	bis in die	twice a day
t.i.d.	ter in die	three times a day
t.d.s.	ter die sumendum	three times a day
q.i.d	quarter in die	four times a day
stat.	statim	immediately
s.o.s.	si opus sit	whenever required
o.m.	omni mane	every morning
o.n.	omni nocte	every night
h.s.	hora somni	at bedtime
rep	repetatur	let it be repeated

B. Routes of Administration

Short form	Full Form
SC	subcutaneous route
IM	intramuscular route
IV	intravenous route
SL	sublingual route
IA	intraarterial route
SD	subdural route
ED	epidural route
PO	per os (by mouth)
PR	per rectum (rectal route)
PV	per vaginam (vaginal route)
BOL	bolus (as a large single dose usually IV)

WEIGHTS AND MEASURES

Decimal system (metric system) is usually used worldwide for scientific work because calculations are very easy and there is direct relation between unit of weights and volume. In this system base for weight is kilogram (kg) and base for volume is litre (l). Solid substances are usually weighed and liquids measured by volume.

Measurement of weight (mass) in metric system	Approximate household measures
1000 femtograms (fg) = 1 picogram (pg)	1 drop = 0.06 ml
1000 picograms (pg) = 1 nanogram (ng)	16 drops = 1 ml
1 microgram = 1000 nanograms (ng)	1Tea spoonful = 5 ml
1 nanogram (ng) = 0.001 microgram (μg/mcg)	1 Dessert spoonful = 10 ml
1000 micrograms (μg/mcg) = 1 milligram (mg)	1 Table spoonful = 15 ml
1000 milligrams (mg) = 1 gram (G/g)	1 Wine glass full = 60 ml
1000 grams (g) = 1 kilogram (kg)	1 Tea cup full = 120 ml
Measurement of capacity (volume) in metric system	1 Tumbler full = 240 ml.
1000 microlitres (μl) = 1 millilitre (ml)	
1000 millilitres (ml) = 1 litre (L)	
1000 litres (L) = 1 kilolitres (Kl)	

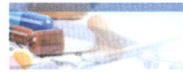

National List of Essential Medicines 2015
(Available from: https://www.nhp.gov.in/essential-drugs_mtl)

Section 1: Anesthetic agents

1.1 General Anesthetics and oxygen

1.1.1	Halothane	S,T	Inhalation
1.1.2	Isoflurane	S,T	Inhalation
1.1.3	Ketamine	P,S,T	Injection 50 mg/ml
1.1.4	Nitrous oxide	P,S,T	Inhalation
1.1.5	Oxygen	P,S,T	Inhalation (Medicinal gas)
1.1.6	Propofol	P,S,T	Injection 10 mg/ml
1.1.7	Sevoflurane	T	Inhalation
1.1.8	Thiopentone	P,S,T	Powder for Injection 0.5 g Powder for Injection 1 g

1.2 Local anesthetics

1.2.1	Bupivacaine	S,T	Injection 0.25% Injection 0.5% Injection 0.5% with 7.5% glucose
1.2.2	Lignocaine	P,S,T	Topical forms 2–5% Injection 1% Injection 2% Injection 5% with 7.5% Glucose
1.2.3	Lignocaine (A) + Adrenaline (B)	P,S,T	Injection 1% (A) + 1:200000 (5 mcg/ml) (B) Injection 2% (A) + 1:200000 (5 mcg/ml) (B)
1.2.4	Prilocaine (A) + Lignocaine (B)	T	Cream 2.5% (A) + 2.5% (B)

1.3 Preoperative medication and sedation for short-term procedures

1.3.1	Atropine	P,S,T	Injection 0.6 mg/ml
1.3.2	Glycopyrrolate	S,T	Injection 0.2 mg/ml
1.3.3	Midazolam	P,S,T	Tablet 7.5 mg Tablet 15 mg Oral liquid 2 mg/ml Injection 1 mg/ml Injection 5 mg/ml
1.3.4	Morphine	P,S,T	Injection 10 mg/ml Injection 15 mg/ml

Section 2: Analgesics, antipyretics, non steroidal anti-inflammatory medicines, medicines used to treat gout and disease modifying agents used in rheumatoid disorders

2.1 Non-opioid analgesics, antipyretics and nonsteroidal anti-inflammatory medicines

2.1.1	Acetylsalicylic acid	P,S,T	Tablet 300 mg to 500 mg Effervescent/Dispersible/Enteric coated Tablet 300 mg to 500 mg
2.1.2	Diclofenac	P,S,T	Tablet 50 mg Injection 25 mg/ml
2.1.3	Ibuprofen	P,S,T	Tablet 200 mg Tablet 400 mg Oral liquid 100 mg/5 ml
2.1.4	Mefenamic acid	P,S,T	Capsule 250 mg Capsule 500 mg Oral liquid 100 mg/5 ml
2.1.5	Paracetamol	P,S,T	Tablet 500 mg Tablet 650 mg All licenced oral liquid dosage forms and strengths Injection 150 mg/ml Suppository 80 mg Suppository 170 mg

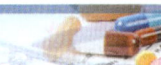

2.2 Opioid analgesics

2.2.1	Fentanyl	S,T	Injection 50 mcg/ml
2.2.2	Morphine	P,S,T	Tablet 10 mg
			Injection 10 mg/ml
			Injection 15 mg/ml
2.2.3	Tramadol	S,T	Capsule 50 mg
			Capsule 100 mg
			Injection 50 mg/ml

2.3 Medicines used to treat gout

2.3.1	Allopurinol	P,S,T	Tablet 100 mg
			Tablet 300 mg
2.3.2	Colchicine	P,S,T	Tablet 0.5 mg

2.4 Disease modifying agents used in rheumatoid disorders

2.4.1	Azathioprine	S, T	Tablet 50 mg
2.4.2	Hydroxychloroquine	S,T	Tablet 200 mg
			Tablet 400 mg
2.4.3	Leflunomide	S,T	Tablet 10 mg
			Tablet 20 mg
2.4.4	Methotrexate	S,T	Tablet 5 mg
			Tablet 7.5 mg
			Tablet 10 mg Injection 25 mg/ ml
2.4.5	Sulfasalazine	S,T	Tablet 500 mg

Section 3: Antiallergics and medicines used in anaphylaxis

3.1	Adrenaline	P,S,T	Injection 1 mg/ml
3.2	Cetirizine	P,S,T	Tablet 10 mg
			Oral liquid 5 mg/5 ml
3.3	Chlorpheniramine	P,S,T	Tablet 4 mg
			Oral liquid 2 mg/5 ml
3.4	Dexamethasone	P,S,T	Tablet 0.5 mg
			Injection 4 mg/ml
3.5	Hydrocortisone	P,S,T	Powder for Injection 100 mg
3.6	Pheniramine	P,S,T	Injection 22.75 mg/ml
3.7	Prednisolone	P,S,T	Tablet 5 mg
			Tablet 10 mg
			Tablet 20 mg
			Oral liquid 5 mg/5 ml
			Oral liquid 15 mg/5 ml

Section 4: Antidotes and other substances used in poisoning

4.1 Nonspecific

4.1.1	Activated charcoal	P,S,T	Powder (as licensed)

4.2 Specific

4.2.1	Atropine	P,S,T	Injection 1 mg/ml
4.2.2	Calcium gluconate	P,S,T	Injection 100 mg/ml
4.2.3	Desferrioxamine	S,T	Powder for Injection 500 mg
4.2.4	Dimercaprol	S,T	Injection 50 mg/ml
4.2.5	Methylthioninium chloride (Methylene blue)	S,T	Injection 10 mg/ml
4.2.6	N-acetylcysteine	P,S,T	Sachet 200 mg
			Injection 200 mg/ml
4.2.7	Naloxone	P,S,T	Injection 0.4 mg/ml
4.2.8	Neostigmine	P,S,T	Injection 0.5 mg/ml

4.2.9	Penicillamine	S,T	Capsule 250 mg
4.2.10	Pralidoxime chloride (2-PAM)	P,S,T	Injection 25 mg/ml
4.2.11	Snake venom antiserum	P,S,T	Injection
	Soluble/liquid polyvalent		Powder for Injection
	Lyophilized polyvalent		
4.2.12	Sodium nitrite	S,T	Injection 30 mg/ml
4.2.13	Sodium thiosulphate	S,T	Injection 100 mg/ml

Section 5: Anticonvulsants/Antiepileptics

5.1	Carbamazepine	P,S,T	Tablet 100 mg
			Tablet 200 mg
			CR Tablet 200 mg
			Tablet 400 mg
			CR Tablet 400 mg
			Oral liquid 100 mg/5 ml
			Oral liquid 200 mg/5 ml
5.2	Clobazam	S,T	Tablet 5 mg
			Tablet 10 mg
5.3	Diazepam	P,S,T	Oral liquid 2 mg/5 ml Injection 5 mg/ml
			Suppository 5 mg
5.4	Levetiracetam	S,T	Tablet 250 mg
			Tablet 500 mg
			Tablet 750 mg
			ER Tablet 750 mg
			Oral liquid 100 mg/ml Injection 100 mg/ml
5.5	Lorazepam	P,S,T	Tablet 1 mg
			Tablet 2 mg
			Injection 2 mg/ml
5.6	Magnesium sulphate	S,T	Injection 500 mg/ml
5.7	Phenobarbitone	P,S,T	Tablet 30 mg
			Tablet 60 mg
			Oral liquid 20 mg/5 ml
		S,T	Injection 200 mg/ml
5.8	Phenytoin	P,S,T	Tablet 50 mg
			Tablet 100 mg
			Tablet 300 mg
			ER Tablet 300 mg
			Oral liquid 30 mg/5 ml
			Oral liquid 125 mg/5 ml
			Injection 25 mg/ml
			Injection 50 mg/ml
5.9	Sodium valproate	P,S,T	Tablet 200 mg
			Tablet 300 mg
			CR Tablet 300 mg
			Tablet 500 mg
			CR Tablet 500 mg
			Oral liquid 200 mg/5ml
		T	Injection 100 mg/ml

Section 6: Anti-infective medicines

6.1 Anthelminthics
6.1.1 Intestinal anthelminthics

6.1.1.1	Albendazole	P,S,T	Tablet 400 mg
			Oral liquid 200 mg/5 ml
6.1.1.2	Mebendazole	P,S,T	Tablet 100 mg
			Oral liquid 100 mg/5 ml

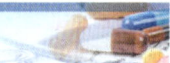

6.1.2 Antifilarial

6.1.2.1	Diethylcarbamazine	P,S,T	Tablet 50 mg Tablet 100 mg Oral liquid 120 mg/5 ml

6.1.3 Anti-schistosomal and anti-trematodal medicine

6.1.3.1	Praziquantel	S,T	Tablet 600 mg

6.2 Antibacterials
6.2.1 Beta lactam medicines

6.2.1.1	Amoxicillin	P,S,T	Capsule 250 mg Capsule 500 mg Oral liquid 250 mg/5 ml
6.2.1.2	Amoxicillin (A) + Clavulanic acid (B)	P,S,T	Tablet 500 mg (A) + 125 mg (B) Oral liquid 200 mg (A) + 28.5 mg (B)/5 ml Dry Syrup 125 mg (A) + 31.25 (B)/5 ml Powder for Injection 500 mg (A) + 100 mg (B)
		S,T	Powder for Injection 1 g (A) + 200 mg (B)
6.2.1.3	Ampicillin	P,S,T	Powder for Injection 500 mg Powder for Injection 1 g
6.2.1.4	Benzathine benzylpenicillin	P,S,T	Powder for Injection 6 lac units Powder for Injection 12 lac units
6.2.1.5	Benzyl penicillin	P,S,T	Powder for Injection 10 lac units
6.2.1.6	Cefadroxil	P,S,T	Tablet 500 mg Tablet 1 g Oral liquid 125 mg/5 ml
6.2.1.7	Cefazolin	P,S,T	Powder for Injection 500 mg Powder for Injection 1 g
6.2.1.8	Cefixime	S,T	Tablet 200 mg Tablet 400 mg Oral liquid 50 mg/5 ml Oral liquid 100 mg/5 ml
6.2.1.9	Cefotaxime	S,T	Powder for Injection 250 mg Powder for Injection 500 mg Powder for Injection 1 g
6.2.1.10	Ceftazidime	S,T	Powder for Injection 250 mg Powder for Injection 1 g
6.2.1.11	Ceftriaxone	S,T	Powder for Injection 250 mg Powder for Injection 500 mg Powder for Injection 1 g Powder for Injection 2 g
6.2.1.12	Cloxacillin	P,S,T	Capsule 250 mg Capsule 500 mg Oral Liquid 125 mg/5 ml Powder for Injection 250 mg
6.2.1.13	Piperacillin (A) + Tazobactam (B)	T	Powder for Injection 1 g (A) + 125 mg (B) Powder for Injection 2 g (A) + 250 mg (B) Powder for Injection 4 g (A) + 500 mg (B)

6.2.2 Other antibacterials

6.2.2.1	Azithromycin	P,S,T	Tablet 250 mg Tablet 500 mg Oral liquid 200 mg/5 ml Powder for Injection 500 mg
6.2.2.2	Ciprofloxacin	P,S,T	Tablet 250 mg Tablet 500 mg Oral liquid 250 mg/5 ml Injection 200 mg/100 ml

6.2.2.3	Clarithromycin	S,T	Tablet 250 mg
			Tablet 500 mg
			Oral liquid 125 mg/5 ml
6.2.2.4	Cotrimoxazole [Sulphamethoxazole (A) + Trimethoprim (B)]	P,S,T	Tablet 400 mg (A) + 80 mg (B)
			Tablet 800 mg (A) + 160 mg (B)
			Oral liquid 200 mg (A) + 40 mg (B)/5 ml
6.2.2.5	Doxycycline	P,S,T	Capsule 100 mg
			Dry Syrup 50 mg/5 ml
6.2.2.6	Gentamicin	P,S,T	Injection 10 mg/ml
			Injection 40 mg/ml
6.2.2.7	Metronidazole	P,S,T	Tablet 200 mg
			Tablet 400 mg
			Oral liquid 200 mg/5 ml
			Injection 500 mg/100 ml
6.2.2.8	Nitrofurantoin	P,S,T	Tablet 100 mg
			Oral liquid 25 mg/5 ml
6.2.2.9	Vancomycin	T	Powder for Injection 250 mg
			Powder for Injection 500 mg
			Powder for Injection 1 g

6.2.3 Antileprosy medicines

6.2.3.1	Clofazimine	P,S,T	Capsule 50 mg
			Capsule 100 mg
6.2.3.2	Dapsone	P,S,T	Tablet 25 mg
			Tablet 50 mg
			Tablet 100 mg
6.2.3.3	Rifampicin	P,S,T	Capsule 150 mg
			Capsule 300 mg

6.2.4 Antituberculosis medicines

6.2.4.1	Capreomycin	P, S, T	Powder for Injection 1 g
6.2.4.2	Cycloserine	P, S, T	Capsule 125 mg
			Capsule 250 mg
6.2.4.3	Ethambutol	P,S,T	Tablet 200 mg
			Tablet 400 mg
			Tablet 600 mg
			Tablet 800 mg
6.2.4.4	Ethionamide	P, S, T	Tablet 125 mg
			Tablet 250 mg
6.2.4.5	Isoniazid	P,S,T	Tablet 50 mg
			Tablet 100 mg
			Tablet 300 mg
			Oral liquid 100 mg/5 ml
6.2.4.6	Kanamycin	P, S, T	Powder for Injection 500 mg
			Powder for Injection 750 mg
			Powder for Injection 1 g
6.2.4.7	Levofloxacin	P, S, T	Tablet 250 mg
			Tablet 500 mg
			Tablet 750 mg
6.2.4.8	Linezolid	P, S, T	Tablet 600 mg
6.2.4.9	Moxifloxacin	P, S, T	Tablet 200 mg
			Tablet 400 mg
6.2.4.10	Para-aminosalicylic acid	P,S,T	Tablet 500 mg Granules (As licensed)
6.2.4.11	Pyrazinamide	P,S,T	Tablet 500 mg
			Tablet 750 mg
			Tablet 1000 mg
			Tablet 1500 mg
			Oral liquid 250 mg/5 ml

6.2.4.12	Rifabutin	S,T	Capsule 150 mg
6.2.4.13	Rifampicin	P,S,T	Capsule 150 mg
			Capsule 300 mg
			Capsule 450 mg
			Capsule 600 mg
			Oral liquid 100 mg/5 ml
6.2.4.14	Streptomycin	P,S,T	Powder for Injection 750 mg
			Powder for Injection 1 g

6.3 Antifungal medicines

6.3.1	Amphotericin B (a) Amphotericin B (conventional) (b) Lipid/Liposomal Amphotericin B	S,T	Powder for Injection 50 mg
6.3.2	Clotrimazole	P,S,T	Pessary 100 mg
6.3.3	Fluconazole	P,S,T	Tablet 100 mg
			Tablet 150 mg
			Tablet 200 mg
			Tablet 400 mg
			Oral liquid 50 mg/5 ml
		S,T	Injection 200 mg /100 ml
6.3.4	Griseofulvin	P,S,T	Tablet 125 mg
			Tablet 250 mg
			Tablet 375 mg
6.3.5	Nystatin	P,S,T	Tablet 500,000 IU
			Pessary 100,000 IU
			Oral Liquid 100, 000 IU/ml

6.4 Antiviral medicines
6.4.1 Antiherpes medicines

6.4.1.1	Acyclovir	P,S,T	Tablet 200 mg
			Tablet 400 mg
			Powder for Injection 250 mg
			Powder for Injection 500 mg
			Oral liquid 400 mg/5 ml

6.4.2 Anti cytomegalovirus (CMV) medicines

6.4.2.1	Ganciclovir	S,T	Capsule 250 mg
			Powder for Injection 500 mg

6.4.3 Antiretroviral medicines
6.4.3.1 Nucleoside reverse transcriptase inhibitors

6.4.3.1.1	Abacavir	S,T	Tablet 60 mg
			Tablet 300 mg
6.4.3.1.2	Abacavir (A) + Lamivudine (B)	S,T	Tablet 60 mg (A) + 30 mg (B) Tablet 600 mg (A) + 300 mg (B)
6.4.3.1.3	Lamivudine (A) + Nevirapine (B) + Stavudine (C)	S,T	Dispersible Tablet 30 mg (A) + 50 mg (B) + 6 mg (C) Tablet 150 mg (A) + 200 mg (B) + 30 mg (C)
6.4.3.1.4	Lamivudine (A) + Zidovudine (B)	S,T	Tablet 30 mg (A) + 60 mg (B) Tablet 150 mg (A) + 300 mg (B)
6.4.3.1.5	Stavudine (A) + Lamivudine (B)	S,T	Dispersible Tablet 6 mg (A) + 30 mg (B) Tablet 30 mg (A) + 150 mg (B)
6.4.3.1.6	Tenofovir (A) + Lamivudine (B)	S,T	Tablet 300 mg (A) + 300 mg (B)
6.4.3.1.7	Tenofovir (A) + Lamivudine (B) + Efavirenz (C)	S,T	Tablet 300 mg (A) + 300 mg (B) + 600 mg (C)
6.4.3.1.8	Zidovudine	S,T	Tablet 300 mg Oral liquid 50 mg/5 ml
6.4.3.1.9	Zidovudine (A) + Lamivudine (B) + Nevirapine (C)	S,T	Tablet 60 mg (A) + 30 mg (B) + 50 mg (C) Tablet 300 mg (A) + 150 mg (B) + 200 mg (C)

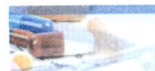

6.4.3.2 Non-nucleoside reverse transcriptase inhibitors

6.4.3.2.1	Efavirenz	S,T	Tablet 50 mg
			Tablet 200 mg
			Tablet 600 mg
6.4.3.2.2	Nevirapine	S,T	Dispersible Tablet 50 mg
			Tablet 200 mg
			Oral liquid 50 mg/5 ml

6.4.3.3 Integrase inhibitors

6.4.3.3.1	Raltegravir	S,T	Tablet 400 mg

6.4.3.4 Protease inhibitors

6.4.3.4.1	Atazanavir (A) + Ritonavir (B)	S,T	Tablet 300 mg (A) + 100 mg (B)
6.4.3.4.2	Darunavir	S,T	Tablet 600 mg
6.4.3.4.3	Lopinavir (A) + Ritonavir (B)	S,T	Tablet 100 mg (A) + 25 mg (B)
			Tablet 200 mg (A) + 50 mg (B)
			Oral liquid 400 mg (A) + 100 mg (B)/ 5ml
6.4.3.4.4	Ritonavir	S,T	Tablet 100 mg

6.4.4 Medicines for hepatitis B and hepatitis C

6.4.4.1	Entecavir	S,T	Tablet 0.5 mg
			Tablet 1 mg
6.4.4.2	Pegylated interferon alfa 2a	S,T	Injection 180 mcg
			Injection 80 mcg
	Pegylated interferon alfa 2b	S,T	Injection 100 mcg
			Injection 120 mcg
6.4.4.3	Ribavirin	S,T	Capsule 200 mg
6.4.4.4	Sofosbuvir	S,T	Tablet 400 mg
6.4.4.5	Tenofovir	S,T	Tablet 300 mg

6.5: Antiprotozoal medicines
6.5.1 Antiamoebic and antigiardiasis medicines

6.5.1.1	Diloxanide furoate	P,S,T	Tablet 500 mg
6.5.1.2	Metronidazole	P,S,T	Tablet 200 mg
			Tablet 400 mg
			Injection 500 mg/100 ml
			Oral liquid 200 mg/5 ml

6.5.2 Antileishmaniasis medicines

6.5.2.1	Amphotericin B	S,T	Powder for Injection 50 mg
	(a) Amphotericin B (conventional)		
	(b) Lipid/Liposomal Amphotericin B		
6.5.2.2	Miltefosine	P,S,T	Capsule 10 mg
			Capsule 50 mg
6.5.2.3	Paromomycin	P,S,T	Injection 375 mg/ml

6.5.3 Antimalarial medicines
6.5.3.1 For curative treatment

6.5.3.1.1	Artemether (A) + Lumefantrine (B)	P,S,T	Tablet 20 mg (A) + 120 mg (B)
			Tablet 40 mg (A) + 240 mg (B)
			Tablet 80 mg (A) + 480 mg (B)
			Oral liquid 80 mg (A) + 480 mg (B)/5 ml
6.5.3.1.2	Artesunate	P,S,T	Powder for Injection 60 mg
			Powder for Injection 120 mg

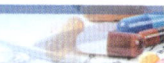

6.5.3.1.3	Artesunate (A) + Sulphadoxine - Pyrimethamine (B)	P,S,T	Combi pack (A+B) 1 Tablet 25 mg (A) + 1 Tablet (250 mg + 12.5 mg) (B) 1 Tablet 50 mg (A) + 1 Tablet (500 mg + 25 mg) (B) 1 Tablet 100 mg (A) + 1 Tablet (750 mg + 37.5 mg) (B) 1 Tablet 150 mg (A) + 2 Tablet (500 mg + 25 mg) (B) 1 Tablet 200 mg (A) + 2 Tablet (750 mg + 37.5 mg) (B)
6.5.3.1.4	Chloroquine	P,S,T	Tablet 150 mg Oral liquid 50 mg/5 ml
6.5.3.1.5	Clindamycin	P,S,T	Capsule 150 mg Capsule 300 mg
6.5.3.1.6	Primaquine	P,S,T	Tablet 2.5 mg Tablet 7.5 mg Tablet 15 mg
6.5.3.1.7	Quinine	P,S,T	Tablet 300 mg Injection 300 mg/ml

6.5.3.2 For prophylaxis

6.5.3.2.1	Mefloquine	T	Tablet 250 mg *Only for use as chemoprophylaxis for long-term travellers like military and travel troops, travelling from low endemic to high endemic area.

6.5.4 Antipneumocystosis and antitoxoplasmosis medicines

6.5.4.1	Cotrimoxazole [Sulphamethoxazole (A) + Trimethoprim (B)]	P,S,T	Tablet 400 mg (A) + 80 mg (B) Tablet 800 mg (A) + 160 mg (B) Oral liquid 200 mg (A) + 40 mg (B)/5 ml
6.5.4.2	Pentamidine	S,T	Powder for Injection 200 mg

Section 7: Antimigraine medicines

7.1.1	Acetylsalicylic acid	P,S,T	Tablet 300 mg to 500 mg Effervescent/Dispersible/Enteric coated Tablet 300 mg to 500 mg
7.1.2	Paracetamol	P,S,T	Tablet 500 mg Tablet 650 mg
7.1.3	Sumatriptan	P,S,T	Tablet 25 mg Tablet 50 mg Injection 6 mg/0.5 ml

7.2 For prophylaxis

7.2.1	Flunarizine	P,S,T	Tablet 5 mg Tablet 10 mg
7.2.2	Propranolol	P,S,T	Tablet 10 mg Tablet 40 mg Tablet 80 mg

Section 8: Antineoplastic/immunosuppressives and medicines used in palliative care

8.1 Antineoplastic medicines

8.1.1	5-Fluorouracil	T	Injection 250 mg/5 ml
8.1.2	6-Mercaptopurine	T	Tablet 50 mg
8.1.3	Actinomycin D	T	Powder for Injection 0.5 mg
8.1.4	All-trans retinoic acid	T	Capsule 10 mg
8.1.5	Arsenic trioxide	T	Injection 1 mg/ml

8.1.6	Bleomycin	T	Powder for Injection 15 units
8.1.7	Bortezomib	T	Powder for Injection 2 mg
8.1.8	Calcium folinate	T	Tablet 15 mg
			Injection 3 mg/ml
8.1.9	Capecitabine	T	Tablet 500 mg
8.1.10	Carboplatin	T	Injection 10 mg/ml
8.1.11	Chlorambucil	T	Tablet 2 mg
			Tablet 5 mg
8.1.12	Cisplatin	T	Injection 1 mg/ml
8.1.13	Cyclophosphamide	T	Tablet 50 mg
			Tablet 200 mg
			Powder for Injection 500 mg
8.1.14	Cytosine arabinoside	T	Injection 100 mg/ml
			Powder for Injection 500 mg
			Powder for Injection 1000 mg
8.1.15	Dacarbazine	T	Powder for Injection 500 mg
			Powder for Injection 200 mg
8.1.16	Daunorubicin	T	Injection 5 mg/ml
8.1.17	Docetaxel	T	Powder for Injection 20 mg
			Powder for Injection 80 mg
8.1.18	Doxorubicin	T	Injection 2 mg/ml
8.1.19	Etoposide	T	Capsule 100 mg
			Injection 20 mg/ml
8.1.20	Gefitinib	T	Tablet 250 mg
8.1.21	Gemcitabine	T	Powder for Injection 200 mg
			Powder for Injection 1 g
8.1.22	Ifosfamide	T	Powder for Injection 1 g
			Powder for Injection 2 g
8.1.23	Imatinib	T	Tablet 100 mg
			Tablet 400 mg
8.1.24	L-Asparaginase	T	Powder for Injection 5000 KU
			Powder for Injection 10000 KU
8.1.25	Melphalan	T	Tablet 2 mg
			Tablet 5 mg
8.1.26	Mesna	T	Injection 100 mg/ml
8.1.27	Methotrexate	T	Tablet 2.5 mg
			Tablet 5 mg
			Tablet 10 mg
			Injection 50 mg/ml
8.1.28	Oxaliplatin	T	Injection 5 mg/ml
8.1.29	Paclitaxel	T	Injection 30 mg/5 ml
			Injection 100 mg/16.7 ml
8.1.30	Procarbazine	T	Capsule 50 mg
8.1.31	Rituximab	T	Injection 10 mg/ml
8.1.32	Temozolomide	T	Capsule 20 mg
			Capsule 100 mg
			Capsule 250 mg
8.1.33	Thalidomide	T	Capsule 50 mg
			Capsule 100 mg
8.1.34	Trastuzumab	T	Injection 440 mg/50 ml
8.1.35	Vinblastine	T	Injection 1 mg/ml
8.1.36	Vincristine	T	Injection 1 mg/ml

8.2 Hormones and antihormones used in cancer therapy

8.2.1	Bicalutamide	T	Tablet 50 mg
8.2.2	Letrozole	T	Tablet 2.5 mg

8.2.3	Prednisolone	S, T	Tablet 10 mg
			Tablet 20 mg
			Tablet 40 mg
			Oral liquid 5 mg/5 ml
			Oral liquid 15 mg/5 ml
			Injection 20 mg/2 ml
8.2.4	Tamoxifen	T	Tablet 10 mg
			Tablet 20 mg

8.3 Immunosuppressive medicines

8.3.1	Azathioprine	T	Tablet 50 mg
8.3.2	Cyclosporine	T	Capsule 10 mg
			Capsule 25 mg
			Capsule 50 mg
			Capsule 100 mg
			Oral liquid 100 mg/ml
			Injection 50 mg/ml
8.3.3	Mycophenolate mofetil	T	Tablet 250 mg
			Tablet 500 mg
8.3.4	Tacrolimus	T	Capsule 0.5 mg
			Capsule 1 mg
			Capsule 2 mg

8.4 Medicines used in palliative care

8.4.1	Allopurinol	T	Tablet 100 mg
8.4.2	Amitriptyline	T	Tablet 10 mg
			Tablet 25 mg
8.4.3	Dexamethasone	T	Tablet 0.5 mg
			Injection 4 mg/ml
8.4.4	Diazepam	T	Tablet 2 mg
			Tablet 5 mg
			Injection 5 mg/ml
8.4.5	Filgrastim	T	Injection 300 mcg
8.4.6	Fluoxetine	T	Capsule 20 mg
8.4.7	Haloperidol	T	Tablet 1.5 mg
			Tablet 5 mg
			Injection 5 mg/ml
8.4.8	Lactulose	T	Oral liquid 10 g/15 ml
8.4.9	Loperamide	T	Tablet 2 mg
8.4.10	Metoclopramide	T	Tablet 10 mg
			Oral liquid 5 mg/5 ml
			Injection 5 mg/ml
8.4.11	Midazolam	T	Injection 1 mg/ml
8.4.12	Morphine	T	Tablet 10 mg
			Tablet 20 mg
			SR Tablet 30 mg
8.4.13	Ondansetron	S,T	Tablet 4 mg
			Tablet 8 mg
			Oral liquid 2 mg/5 ml
			Injection 2 mg/ml
8.4.14	Tramadol	T	Capsule 50 mg
			Capsule 100 mg
			Injection 50 mg/ml
8.4.15	Zoledronic acid	T	Powder for Injection 4 mg

Section 9: Antiparkinsonism medicines

9.1	Levodopa (A) + Carbidopa (B)	P,S,T	Tablet 100 mg (A) + 10 mg (B)
			Tablet 100 mg (A) + 25 mg (B)
			CR Tablet 100 mg (A) + 25 mg (B)
			CR Tablet 200 mg (A) + 50 (B) mg
			Tablet 250 mg (A) + 25 mg (B)
9.2	Trihexyphenidyl	P,S,T	Tablet 2 mg

Section 10: Medicines affecting blood

10.1 Antianaemia medicines

10.1.1	Erythropoietin	S,T	Injection 2000 IU/ml
			Injection 10000 IU/ml
10.1.2	Ferrous salts	P,S,T	Tablet equivalent to 60 mg of elemental iron
			Oral liquid equivalent to 25 mg of elemental iron/ml
10.1.3	Ferrous salt (A) + Folic acid (B)	P,S,T	Tablet 45 mg elemental iron (A) + 400 mcg (B)
			Tablet 100 mg elemental iron (A) + 500 mcg (B)
			Oral liqiud 20 mg elemental iron (A) + 100 mcg (B)/ml
10.1.4	Folic acid	P,S,T	Tablet 5 mg
10.1.5	Hydroxocobalamin	P,S,T	Injection 1 mg/ml
10.1.6	Hydroxyurea	P,S,T	Capsule 500 mg
10.1.7	Iron sucrose	S,T	Injection 20 mg/ml

10.2 Medicines affecting coagulation

10.2.1	Enoxaparin	T	Injection 40 mg/0.4 ml
			Injection 60 mg/0.6 ml
10.2.2	Heparin	S,T	Injection 1000 IU/ml
			Injection 5000 IU/ml
10.2.3	Phytomenadione (Vitamin K_1)	P,S,T	Tablet 10 mg
			Injection 10 mg/ml
10.2.4	Protamine	S,T	Injection 10 mg/ml
10.2.5	Tranexamic acid	P,S,T	Tablet 500 mg
			Injection 100 mg/ml
10.2.6	Warfarin	S,T	Tablet 1 mg
			Tablet 2 mg
			Tablet 3 mg
			Tablet 5 mg

Section 11: Blood products and Plasma substitutes

11.1 Blood and Blood components

All forms of the following as approved by licensing authority are considered as included in NLEM. However, considering the process, technology and other relevant aspects, they should be considered differently for purposes such as procurement policy, pricing, etc.

11.1.1	Fresh frozen plasma	S,T	As licensed
11.1.2	Platelet rich plasma	S,T	As licensed
11.1.3	Red blood cells	S,T	As licensed
11.1.4	Whole blood	S,T	As licensed

11.2 Plasma substitutes

| 11.2.1 | Dextran-40 | S,T | Injection 10% |

11.3 Plasma fractions for specific use

In case of coagulation factors and other blood products, irrespective of variation in source, all forms of these products as approved by licensing authority are considered as included in NLEM. However, considering the source, process, technology and other relevant aspects, they should be considered differently for purposes such as procurement policy, pricing, etc.

11.3.1	Coagulation factor IX	S,T	Powder for Injection 600 IU
11.3.2	Coagulation factor VIII	S,T	Powder for Injection 250 IU
			Powder for Injection 500 IU
11.3.3	Cryoprecipitate	S,T	As licensed

Section 12: Cardiovascular medicines

12.1 Medicines used in angina

12.1.1	Acetylsalicylic acid	P,S,T	Tablet 75 mg
			Effervescent/Dispersible/Enteric coated Tablet 75 mg
			Tablet 100 mg
			Effervescent/Dispersible/Enteric coated Tablet 100 mg
			Tablet 150 mg
			Effervescent/Dispersible/Enteric coated Tablet 150 mg
12.1.2	Clopidogrel	P,S,T	Tablet 75 mg
12.1.3	Diltiazem	P,S,T	Tablet 30 mg
			Tablet 60 mg
			SR Tablet 90 mg
		T	Injection 5 mg/ml
12.1.4	Glyceryl trinitrate	P,S,T	Sublingual tablet 0.5 mg
		S,T	Injection 5 mg/ml
12.1.5	Isosorbide-5-mononitrate	P,S,T	Tablet 10 mg
			Tablet 20 mg
			SR Tablet 30 mg
			SR Tablet 60 mg
12.1.6	Isosorbide dinitrate	P,S,T	Tablet 5 mg
			Tablet 10 mg
12.1.7	Metoprolol	P,S,T	Tablet 25 mg
			Tablet 50 mg
			SR Tablet 25 mg
			SR Tablet 50 mg

12.2 Antiarrhythmic medicines

12.2.1	Adenosine	S,T	Injection 3 mg/ml
12.2.2	Amiodarone	S,T	Tablet 100 mg
			Tablet 200 mg
			Injection 50 mg/ml
12.2.3	Esmolol	T	Injection 10 mg/ml
12.2.4	Lignocaine	S,T	Injection 2% (Preservative free for IV use)
12.2.5	Verapamil	S,T	Tablet 40 mg
			Tablet 80 mg
			Injection 2.5 mg/ml

12.3 Antihypertensive medicines

12.3.1	Amlodipine	P,S,T	Tablet 2.5 mg
			Tablet 5 mg
			Tablet 10 mg
12.3.2	Atenolol	P,S,T	Tablet 50 mg
			Tablet 100 mg
12.3.3	Enalapril	P,S,T	Tablet 2.5 mg
			Tablet 5 mg
12.3.4	Hydrochlorothiazide	P,S,T	Tablet 12.5 mg
			Tablet 25 mg
12.3.5	Labetalol	P,S,T	Injection 5 mg/ml
12.3.6	Methyldopa	P,S,T	Tablet 250 mg
			Tablet 500 mg
12.3.7	Ramipril	P,S,T	Tablet 2.5 mg
			Tablet 5 mg

12.3.8	Sodium nitroprusside	T	Injection 10 mg/ml
12.3.9	Telmisartan	P,S,T	Tablet 20 mg
			Tablet 40 mg
			Tablet 80 mg

12.4 Medicines used in shock and heart failure

12.4.1	Digoxin	S,T	Tablet 0.25 mg
			Oral liquid 0.05 mg/ml
			Injection 0.25 mg/ml
12.4.2	Dobutamine	S,T	Injection 50 mg/ml
12.4.3	Dopamine	S,T	Injection 40 mg/ml
12.4.4	Noradrenaline	S,T	Injection 2 mg/ml

12.5 Antithrombotic medicine (Cardiovascular/ Cerebrovascular)

12.5.1	Acetylsalicylic acid	P,S,T	Tablet 75 mg
			Effervescent/Dispersible/Enteric coated Tablet 75 mg
			Tablet 100 mg
			Acetylsalicylic acid
			Effervescent/Dispersible/Enteric coated Tablet 100 mg
			Tablet 150 mg
			Effervescent/Dispersible/Enteric coated Tablet 150 mg
12.5.2	Alteplase	T	Powder for Injection 20 mg
			Powder for Injection 50 mg
12.5.3	Heparin	S,T	Injection 1000 IU/ml
			Injection 5000 IU/ml
12.5.4	Streptokinase	S,T	Injection 750,000 IU
			Injection 15,00,000 IU

12.6 Hypolipidemic medicines

12.6.1	Atorvastatin	P,S,T	Tablet 10 mg
			Tablet 20 mg
			Tablet 40 mg

Section 13: Medicines used in dementia

13.1	Donepezil	S,T	Tablet 5 mg
			Tablet 10 mg

Section 14: Dermatological medicines (Topical)

14.1 Antifungal medicines

14.1.1	Clotrimazole	P,S,T	Cream 1%

14.2 Anti-infective medicines

14.2.1	Framycetin	P,S,T	Cream 0.5%
14.2.2	Fusidic acid	P,S,T	Cream 2%
14.2.3	Methylrosanilinium chloride (Gentian Violet)	P,S,T	Topial preparation 0.25% to 2%
14.2.4	Povidone iodine	P,S,T	Solution 4% to 10%
14.2.5	Silver sulphadiazine	P,S,T	Cream 1%

14.3 Anti-inflammatory and antipruritic medicines

14.3.1	Betamethasone	P,S,T	Cream 0.05%
			Cream 0.1%
14.3.2	Calamine	P,S,T	Lotion (As per IP)

14.4 Medicines affecting skin differentiation and proliferation

14.4.1	Benzoyl peroxide	P,S,T	Gel 2.5%
14.4.2	Coal tar	P,S,T	Solution 5%

14.4.3	Podophyllin resin	S,T	Solution 10% to 25%
14.4.4	Salicylic acid	P,S,T	Ointment 6%

14.5 Scabicides and pediculicides

			Lotion 1%
14.5.1	Permethrin	P,S,T	Cream 5%

14.6 Miscellaneous

14.6.1	Glycerin	P,S,T	Oral Liquid
14.6.2	White Petrolatum	P,S,T	Jelly 100%

Section 15: Diagnostic agents

15.1 Ophthalmic medicines

15.1.1	Fluorescein	S,T	Eyedrop 1%
15.1.2	Lignocaine	S,T	Eyedrop 4%
15.1.3	Tropicamide	S,T	Eyedrop 1%

15.2 Radiocontrast media

15.2.1	Barium sulphate	S,T	Oral liquid 100% w/v
			Oral liquid 250% w/v
15.2.2	Gadobenate	T	Injection 529 mg/ml
15.2.3	Iohexol	S,T	Injection 140 to 350 mg iodine/ml
15.2.4	Meglumine diatrizoate	S,T	Injection 60% w/v
			Injection 76% w/v

Section 16: Dialysis solutions

16.1	Haemodialysis fluid	S,T	As licensed
16.2	Intraperitoneal dialysis solution	S,T	As licensed

Section 17: Disinfectants and antiseptics

17.1 Antiseptics

17.1.1	Cetrimide	P,S,T	Solution 20% (Concentrate for dilution)
17.1.2	Chlorhexidine	P,S,T	Solution 5% (Concentrate for dilution)
17.1.3	Ethyl alcohol (Denatured)	P,S,T	Solution 70%
17.1.4	Hydrogen peroxide	P,S,T	Solution 6%
17.1.5	Methylrosanilinium chloride (Gentian Violet)	P,S,T	Topial preparation 0.25% to 2%
17.1.6	Povidone iodine	P,S,T	Solution 4% to 10%

17.2 Disinfectants

17.2.1	Bleaching powder	P,S,T	Containing not less than 30% w/w of available chlorine (as per I.P)
17.2.2	Glutaraldehyde	S,T	Solution 2%
17.2.3	Potassium permanganate	P,S,T	Crystals for topical solution

Section 18: Diuretics

18.1	Furosemide	P,S,T	Tablet 40 mg
			Oral liquid 10 mg/ml
			Injection 10 mg/ml
18.2	Hydrochlorothiazide	P,S,T	Tablet 25 mg
			Tablet 50 mg
18.3	Mannitol	P,S,T	Injection 10%
			Injection 20%
18.4	Spironolactone	P,S,T	Tablet 25 mg
			Tablet 50 mg

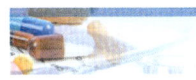

Section 19: Ear, nose and throat medicines			
19.1	Budesonide	P,S,T	Nasal Spray 50 mcg/dose
			Nasal Spray 100 mcg/dose
19.2	Ciprofloxacin	P,S,T	Drops 0.3%
19.3	Clotrimazole	P,S,T	Drops 1%
19.4	Xylometazoline	P,S,T	Nasal drops 0.05 %
			Nasal drops 0.1 %

Section 20: Gastrointestinal medicines			
20.1 Antiulcer medicines			
20.1.1	Omeprazole	P,S,T	Capsule 10 mg
			Capsule 20 mg
			Capsule 40 mg
			Powder for oral liquid 20 mg
20.1.2	Pantoprazole	S,T	Injection 40 mg
20.1.3	Ranitidine	P,S,T	Tablet 150 mg
			Oral liquid 75 mg/5 ml
			Injection 25 mg/ml
20.1.4	Sucralfate	S,T	Oral liquid 1 g
20.2 Antiemetics			
20.2.1	Domperidone	P,S,T	Tablet 10 mg
			Oral liquid 1 mg/ml
20.2.2	Metoclopramide	P,S,T	Injection 5 mg/ml
20.2.3	Ondansetron	S,T	Tablet 4 mg
			Oral liquid 2 mg/5 ml
			Injection 2 mg/ml
20.3 Anti-inflammatory medicines			
20.3.1	5-aminosalicylic acid	S,T	Tablet 400 mg
			Suppository 500 mg Retention Enema
20.4 Antispasmodic medicines			
20.4.1	Dicyclomine	P,S,T	Tablet 10 mg
			Oral solution 10 mg/5 ml Injection 10 mg/ml
20.4.2	Hyoscine butylbromide	P,S,T	Tablet 10 mg
			Injection 20 mg/ml
20.5 Laxatives			
20.5.1	Bisacodyl	P,S,T	Tablet 5 mg
			Suppository 5 mg
20.5.2	Ispaghula	P,S,T	Granules/Husk/Powder
20.5.3	Lactulose	S,T	Oral liquid 10 g/15 ml
20.6 Medicines used in diarrhoea			
20.6.1	Oral rehydration salts	P,S,T	As licensed
20.6.2	Zinc sulphate	P,S,T	Dispersible Tablet 20 mg
20.7 Other medicines			
20.7.1	Somatostatin	T	Powder for Injection 3 mg

Section 21: Hormones, other endocrine medicines and contraceptives			
21.1 Adrenal hormones and synthetic substitutes			
21.1.1	Dexamethasone	S,T	Tablet 0.5 mg
			Injection 4 mg/ml
21.1.2	Human chorionic gonadotropin	T	Injection 1000 IU
			Injection 5000 IU

21.1.3	Hydrocortisone	P,S,T	Tablet 5 mg
			Tablet 10 mg
			Injection 100 mg/ml
21.1.4	Methylprednisolone	S,T	Tablet 8 mg
			Tablet 16 mg
			Tablet 32 mg
			Injection 40 mg/ml
21.1.5	Prednisolone	P,S,T	Tablet 5 mg
			Tablet 10 mg

21.2 Contraceptives
21.2.1 Hormonal contraceptives

| 21.2.1.1 | Ethinylestradiol (A) + Levonorgestrel (B) | P,S,T | Tablet 0.03 mg (A) + 0.15 mg (B) |
| 21.2.1.2 | Ethinylestradiol (A) + Norethisterone (B) | P,S,T | Tablet 0.035 mg (A) + 1 mg (B) |

21.2.2 Intrauterine devices

| 21.2.2.1 | Hormone releasing IUD | T | Contains 52 mg of Levonorgestrel |
| 21.2.2.2 | IUD containing copper | P,S,T | As licensed |

21.2.3 Barrier methods

| 21.2.3.1 | Condom | P,S,T | As per the standards prescribed in Schedule R of Drugs and Cosmetics rules, 1945 |

21.3 Estrogens

21.3.1	Ethinylestradiol	P,S,T	Tablet 0.01 mg
			Tablet 0.05 mg
21.3.2	Levonorgestrel	P,S,T	Tablet 0.75 mg

21.4 Medicines used in diabetes mellitus
21.4.1 Insulins and other antidiabetic agents

21.4.1.1	Glimepiride	P,S,T	Tablet 1 mg
			Tablet 2 mg
21.4.1.2	Insulin (Soluble)	P,S,T	Injection 40 IU/ml
21.4.1.3	Intermediate Acting (NPH) Insulin	P,S,T	Injection 40 IU/ml
			Tablet 500 mg
21.4.1.4	Metformin	P,S,T	Tablet 750 mg
			Tablet 1000 mg
			(Immediate and controlled release)
21.4.1.5	Premix Insulin 30 : 70 Injection (Regular : NPH)	P,S,T	Injection 40 IU/ml

21.4.2 Medicines used to treat hypoglycaemia

| 21.4.2.1 | Glucose | P,S,T | Injection 25 % |

21.5 Ovulation Inducers

| 21.5.1 | Clomiphene | T | Tablet 50 mg |
| | | | Tablet 100 mg |

21.6 Progestogens

21.6.1	Medroxyprogester oneacetate	P,S,T	Tablet 5 mg
			Tablet 10 mg
21.6.2	Norethisterone	P,S,T	Tablet 5 mg

21.7 Thyroid and antithyroid medicines

| 21.7.1 | Carbimazole | P,S,T | Tablet 5 mg |
| | | | Tablet 10 mg |

21.7.2	Levothyroxine	P,S,T	Tablet 12.5 mcg to 150 mcg* (Several strengths are available in market such as 12.5, 25, 50, 62.5, 75, 88, 100, 112 mcg. Therefore it was considered to give a range of available strengths)

Section 22: Immunologicals

In case of these biologicals, irrespective of variation in source, composition and strengths, all the products of the same vaccine/sera/immunoglobulin, as approved by licensing authority are considered as included in NLEM. However, considering the source, process, technology and other relevant aspects, different products of the same biologicals should be considered differently for purposes such as procurement policy, pricing, etc.

22.1 Diagnostic agents

22.1.1	Tuberculin, Purified Protein derivative	P,S,T	

22.2 Sera and immunoglobulins (Liquid/Lyophilized)

22.2.1	Anti-rabies immunoglobulin	P,S,T	
22.2.2	Anti-tetanus immunoglobulin	P,S,T	
22.2.3	Anti-D immunoglobulin	S, T	
22.2.4	Diphtheria antitoxin	P,S,T	
22.2.5	Hepatitis B immunoglobulin	S,T	
22.2.6	Human normal immunoglobulin Snake venom antiserum Soluble/liquid polyvalent	T	
22.2.7	Lyophilized polyvalent	P,S,T	

22.3 Vaccines

(a) All the vaccines which are under Universal Immunization Programme of India (UIP) will be deemed included in NLEM. Presently, the UIP has BCG, DPT, OPV, measles, Hepatitis B, Japanese encephalitis and Pentavalent Vaccines.

(b) The new vaccines, which have been approved by National Technical Advisory Group on Immunization (NTAGI)and planned to be given under UIP, will be deemed to be included as and when listed in UIP. These vaccines are inactivated polio vaccine (IPV), Measles Rubella (MR) and Rotavirus vaccine.

(c) In future, the vaccines which are under consideration, if and when included in UIP, will also be deemed included from the date of inclusion in UIP. These are pneumococcal and HPV vaccines.

22.3.1 For universal immunisation

22.3.1.1	BCG vaccine DPT + Hib + Hep B vaccine	P,S,T	
22.3.1.2		P,S,T	
22.3.1.3	DPT vaccine	P,S,T	
22.3.1.4	Hepatitis B vaccine Japanese encephalitis vaccine	P,S,T	
22.3.1.5		P,S,T	
22.3.1.6	Measles vaccine Oral poliomyelitis vaccine	P,S,T	
22.3.1.7		P,S,T	
22.3.1.8	Tetanus toxoid	P,S,T	

22.3.2 For Specific Group of Individuals

22.3.2.1	Rabies vaccine	P,S,T	

Section 23: Muscle relaxants and cholinesterase inhibitors

23.1	Atracurium	S,T	Injection 10 mg/ml Tablet 5 mg
23.2	Baclofen	S,T	Tablet 10 mg Tablet 20 mg
23.3	Neostigmine	S,T	Tablet 15 mg Injection 0.5 mg/ml

23.4	Succinylcholine	S,T	Injection 50 mg/ml
23.5	Vecuronium	S,T	Powder for Injection 4 mg
			Powder for Injection 10 mg

Section 24: Medicines for neonatal care

24.1	Alprostadil	T	Injection 0.5 mg/ml
24.2	Caffeine	S,T	Oral liquid 20 mg/ml Injection 20 mg/ml
24.3	Surfactant	S,T	Suspension for intratracheal instillation (As licensed)

Section 25: Ophthalmological medicines

25.1 Anti-infective medicine

25.1.1	Acyclovir	P,S,T	Ointment 3%
25.1.2	Ciprofloxacin	P,S,T	Drops 0.3 %
			Ointment 0.3%
25.1.3	Erythromycin	P,S,T	Ointment 0.5%
25.1.4	Gentamicin	P,S,T	Drops 0.3%
25.1.5	Natamycin	P,S,T	Drops 5%
25.1.6	Povidone iodine	P,S,T	Drops 0.6%
			Drops 5%

25.2 Anti-inflammatory medicine

| 25.2.1 | Prednisolone | P,S,T | Drops 0.1% |
| | | | Drops 1% |

25.3 Local anaesthetics

| 25.3.1 | Proparacaine | P,S,T | Drops 0.5% |

25.4 Miotics and antiglaucoma medicines

25.4.1	Acetazolamide	P,S,T	Tablet 250 mg
			Drops 2%
25.4.2	Pilocarpine	P,S,T	Drops 4%
			Drops 0.25%
25.4.3	Timolol	P,S,T	Drops 0.5%

25.5 Mydriatics

25.5.1	Atropine	P,S,T	Drops 1%
			Ointment 1%
25.5.2	Homatropine	P,S,T	Drops 2%
			Drops 5%
25.5.3	Phenylephrine	P,S,T	Drops 10 %
25.5.4	Tropicamide	P,S,T	Drops 1%

25.6 Ophthalmic surgical aids

| 25.6.1 | Hydroxypropyl methylcellulose | T | Injection 2% |

25.7 Miscellaneous

| 25.7.1 | Carboxymethylcellulose | P,S,T | Drops 0.5% |
| | | | Drops 1 % |

Section 26: Oxytocics and antioxytocics

26.1 Oxytocics and abortifacient

26.1.1	Dinoprostone	S,T	Tablet 0.5 mg
			Gel 0.5 mg
26.1.2	Methylergometrine	P,S,T	Tablet 0.125 mg
			Injection 0.2 mg/ml
26.1.3	Mifepristone	T	Tablet 200 mg

26.1.4	Misoprostol	T	Tablet 100 mcg
			Tablet 200 mcg
26.1.5	Oxytocin	S,T	Injection 5 IU/ml
			Injection 10 IU/ml

26.2 Medicines used in preterm labour

| 26.2.1 | Betamethasone | P,S,T | Injection 4 mg/ml |
| 26.2.2 | Nifedipine | S,T | Tablet 10 mg |

Section 27: Psychotherapeutic medicines

27.1 Medicines used in psychotic disorders

27.1.1	Clozapine	T	Tablet 25 mg
			Tablet 50 mg
			Tablet 100 mg
27.1.2	Fluphenazine	S,T	Depot Injection 25 mg/ml
			Tablet 5 mg
			Tablet 10 mg
27.1.3	Haloperidol	S,T	Tablet 20 mg
			Oral liquid 2 mg/5 ml
			Tablet 1 mg
			Tablet 2 mg
27.1.4	Risperidone	P,S,T	Tablet 4 mg
			Oral liquid 1 mg/ml

27.2 Medicines used in mood disorders
27.2.1 Medicines used in depressive disorders

27.2.1.1	Amitriptyline	P,S,T	Tablet 10 mg
			Tablet 25 mg
			Tablet 50 mg
			Tablet 75 mg
			Tablet 5 mg
27.2.1.2	Escitalopram	S,T	Tablet 10 mg
			Tablet 20 mg
			Capsule 10 mg
			Capsule 20 mg
27.2.1.3	Fluoxetine	P,S,T	Capsule 40 mg
			Capsule 60 mg

27.2.2 Medicines used in Bipolar disorders

27.2.2.1	Lithium	S,T	Tablet 300 mg
27.2.2.2	Sodium valproate	P,S,T	Tablet 200 mg
			Tablet 500 mg

27.3 Medicines used for Generalized Anxiety and Sleep Disorders

27.3.1	Clonazepam	P,S,T	Tablet 0.25 mg
			Tablet 0.5 mg
			Tablet 1 mg
27.3.2	Zolpidem	P,S,T	Tablet 5 mg
			Tablet 10 mg

27.4 Medicines used for obsessive compulsive disorders and panic attacks

27.4.1	Clomipramine	S,T	Capsule 10 mg
			Capsule 25 mg
			Capsule 75 mg
27.4.2	Fluoxetine	P,S,T	Capsule 10 mg
			Capsule 20 mg
			Capsule 40 mg
			Capsule 60 mg

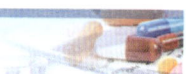

Section 28: Medicines acting on the respiratory tract

28.1 Antiasthmatic medicines

28.1.1	Budesonide	P,S,T	Inhalation (MDI/DPI) 100 mcg/dose
			Inhalation (MDI/DPI) 200 mcg/dose
			Respirator solution for use in nebulizer 0.5 mg/ml
			Respirator solution for use in nebulizer 1 mg/ml
28.1.2	Budesonide (A) + Formoterol (B)	P,S,T	Inhalation (MDI/DPI) 100 mcg (A) + 6 mcg (B)
			Inhalation (MDI/DPI) 200 mcg (A) + 6 mcg (B)
			Inhalation (MDI/DPI) 400 mcg (A) + 6 mcg (B)
28.1.3	Hydrocortisone	P,S,T	Injection 100 mg
			Injection 200 mg
28.1.4	Ipratropium	P,S,T	Inhalation (MDI/DPI) 20 mcg/dose Respirator solution for use in nebulizer 250 mcg/ml
28.1.5	Salbutamol	P,S,T	Tablet 2 mg
			Tablet 4 mg
			Oral liquid 2 mg/5 ml
			Inhalation (MDI/DPI) 100 mcg/dose
			Respirator solution for use in nebulizer 5 mg/ml
28.1.6	Tiotropium	P,S,T	Inhalation (MDI) 9 mcg/dose
			Inhalation (DPI) 18 mcg/dose
			MDI- Metered dose inhaler
			DPI- Dry Powder inhaler

Section 29: Solutions correcting water, electrolyte disturbances and acid–base disturbances

29.1	Glucose	P,S,T	Injection 5%
			Injection 10%
			Injection 25%
			Injection 50%
29.2	Glucose (A) + Sodium chloride (B)	P,S,T	Injection 5% (A) + 0.9% (B)
29.3	Oral rehydration salts	P,S,T	As licensed
29.4	Potassium chloride	P,S,T	Injection 150 mg/ml Oral liquid 500 mg/5 ml
29.5	Ringer lactate	P,S,T	Injection (as per IP)
29.6	Sodium bicarbonate	P,S,T	Injection (as per IP)
29.7	Sodium chloride	P,S,T	Injection 0.9%
			Injection 0.45%
		S,T	Injection 3%

29.3 Miscellaneous

29.3.1	Water for Injection	P,S,T	Injection

Section 30: Vitamins and minerals

30.1	Ascorbic acid (Vitamin C)	P,S,T	Tablet 100 mg
			Tablet 500 mg
30.2	Calcium carbonate	P,S,T	Tablet 250 mg
			Tablet 500 mg
30.3	Calcium gluconate	P,S,T	Injection 100 mg/ml
30.4	Cholecalciferol	P,S,T	Tablet 1000 IU,
			Tablet 60000 IU
			Oral liquid 400 IU/ml

30.5	Nicotinamide	P,S,T	Tablet 50 mg
			Tablet 10 mg
30.6	Pyridoxine	P,S,T	Tablet 50 mg
			Tablet 100 mg
30.7	Riboflavin	P,S,T	Tablet 5 mg
30.8	Thiamine	P,S,T	Tablet 100 mg
			Injection 100 mg/ml
			Capsule 5000 IU
			Capsule 50000 IU
30.9	Vitamin A	P,S,T	Capsule 100000 IU
			Oral liquid 100000 IU/ml
			Injection 50000 IU/ml

P (Primary), S (Secondary), T (Tertiary) health centres.

Logbook

This is to certify that Mr/Ms _____, admitted

in the year _____, in the _____, has satisfactorily completed/

has not completed all assignments mentioned in this Pharmacology logbook for Second Professional MBBS

during the period from _____ to _____ She/ He is / is not eligible to appear for

the summative (University) assessment as on the date given below.

Place:

Date:

_____
Signature of Head of the Department with Seal
(Department of Pharmacology)

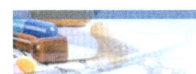

PHARMACOLOGY (PH) CERTIFIABLE COMPETENCIES

Sr. No.	Competency No.	Competency	No. of procedures to be done independently for certification
1.	PH 3.1	Write a rational, correct and legible generic prescription for a given condition and communicate the same to the patient	5
2.	PH 3.2	Perform and interpret a critical appraisal (audit) of a given prescription	3
3.	PH 3.3	Perform a critical evaluation of the drug promotional literature	3
4.	PH 3.5	To prepare and explain a list of P-drugs for a given case/condition	3
5.	PH 3.4	To recognize and report an adverse drug reaction	0
6.	PH 3.6	Demonstrate how to optimize interaction with pharmaceutical representative to get authentic information on drugs	0
7.	PH 3.7	Prepare a list of essential medicines for a healthcare facility	0

Note: In this manual, for certifiable competencies various exercises are given but different exercises can be used to certify that competency.

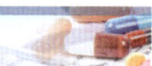

Competency # addressed	Name of activity	Date completed: dd/ mm/yyyy	Attempt at activity First or only (F) Repeat (R) Remedial (Re)	Rating Below (B) expectations Meets (M) expectations Exceeds (E) expectations or numerical score	Decision of faculty Completed (C) Repeat (R) Remedial (Re)	Initial of faculty and date	Feedback received Initial of learner

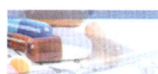

Competency # addressed	Name of activity	Date completed: dd/ mm/yyyy	Attempt at activity First or only (F) Repeat (R) Remedial (Re)	Rating Below (B) expectations Meets (M) expectations Exceeds (E) expectations or numerical score	Decision of faculty Completed (C) Repeat (R) Remedial (Re)	Initial of faculty and date	Feedback received Initial of learner

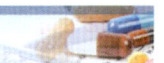

Competency # addressed	Name of activity	Date completed: dd/ mm/yyyy	Attempt at activity First or only (F) Repeat (R) Remedial (Re)	Rating Below (B) expectations Meets (M) expectations Exceeds (E) expectations or numerical score	Decision of faculty Completed (C) Repeat (R) Remedial (Re)	Initial of faculty and date	Feedback received Initial of learner